Praise for *The Ayurvedic Guide to Fertility*

"It's about time we had a book like this one. *The Ayurvedic Guide to Fertility* provides a friendly and honest approach to Ayurveda's wisdom and how modern women can apply it to improve their health before conception. From her research as well as from personal experience, Heather Grzych has created a trustworthy guide into what can be a sensitive topic. Ayurveda is a gold mine for women on the journey to conception, and Heather offers clear and practical guidance to readers. This book is a boon to women!"

— **Kate O'Donnell,** author of *The Everyday Ayurveda Cookbook,*
Ayurveda Cooking for a Calm, Clear Mind, and
The Everyday Ayurveda Guide to Self-Care

"*The Ayurvedic Guide to Fertility* offers a new and refreshing perspective on not just fertility but health for women. This guide is overdue, as it offers an approach that includes rest and self-love — something our current society doesn't always revere but can greatly benefit from."

— **Sarah Kucera,** author of *The Ayurvedic Self-Care Handbook*

"Getting pregnant is a sacred meditation. Heather Grzych has put together essential aspects of fertility in a way that's easy to understand and comfortable to execute. This is a perfect book for all those who are looking to conceive a new life mindfully."

— **Chandresh Bhardwaj,** spiritual adviser and author of
Break the Norms

"Relax and work with nature to conceive a new life for yourself and your family. This is a book I'd be glad to recommend to my treasured clients, as well as my beloved thirtysomething daughter. With nesting, resting, nourishment, and easy-to-experience processes, Heather Grzych draws effectively on the depth and knowledge of her revered mentor, Dr. Sarita Shrestha, Ayurvedic ob-gyn. A must-read."

— **Amadea Morningstar,** author of *The Ayurvedic Cookbook*
and *Easy Healing Drinks from the Wisdom of Ayurveda*

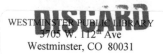

The

AYURVEDIC GUIDE TO FERTILITY

The

AYURVEDIC GUIDE TO FERTILITY

A Natural Approach to Getting Pregnant

HEATHER GRZYCH

Foreword by Dr. John Douillard, DC, CAP

New World Library
Novato, California

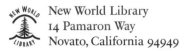

New World Library
14 Pamaron Way
Novato, California 94949

Text design by Tona Pearce Myers

Library of Congress Cataloging-in-Publication Data

Names: Grzych, Heather, date, author.
Title: The ayurvedic guide to fertility : a natural approach to getting pregnant / Heather Grzych.
Description: Novato, California : New World Library, [2020] | Includes bibliographical references and index. | Summary: "A guide to getting pregnant and giving birth to a healthy child using the ancient Indian medical system of Ayurveda, the 'sister science of yoga.' The book covers topics such as adopting an Ayurvedic diet, practicing yoga, cleansing toxins, and creating a healthy environment for conception."-- Provided by publisher.
Identifiers: LCCN 2020002480 (print) | LCCN 2020002481 (ebook) | ISBN 9781608686803 (paperback) | ISBN 9781608686810 (epub)
Subjects: LCSH: Conception--Popular works. | Fertility, Human--Popular works. | Medicine, Ayurvedic--Popular works.
Classification: LCC RG133 .G78 2020 (print) | LCC RG133 (ebook) | DDC 613.9--dc23
LC record available at https://lccn.loc.gov/2020002480
LC ebook record available at https://lccn.loc.gov/2020002481

First printing, May 2020
ISBN 978-1-60868-680-3
Ebook ISBN 978-1-60868-681-0
Printed in the United States on 30% postconsumer-waste recycled paper

New World Library is proud to be a Gold Certified Environmentally Responsible Publisher. Publisher certification awarded by Green Press Initiative.

10   9   8   7   6   5   4   3   2   1

To my son, Gabriel, who came to me in a sleeping dream
and has made my life a waking dream.
And to all the lovers and all the mothers — for staying wild.

Contents

Foreword

As the old saying goes, when the student is ready, the teacher will appear. Thankfully, the teacher, Heather Grzych, has appeared with her book, *The Ayurvedic Guide to Fertility*. The students are ready, and the need is urgent.

I've had many patients come to me for fertility, but one immediately comes to mind: an extremely stressed, high-strung, type A thirty-nine-year-old medical doctor, who demanded she get pregnant within the next three months because after that she had some prescheduled events that she could not miss. She calculated that she had about a four-week window she could take off work in the next year to deliver the baby and then get back to her eighty-hour workweeks. For her plan to work, she had to get pregnant soon. I told her babies have their own schedule and it is impossible and unwise to try to control their arrival. When I proposed revising her plan to include pregnancy preparation, nesting, and dialing down her workload, it only irritated her.

I have been practicing Ayurveda full-time since 1986, and while I do not consider myself a fertility expert, my Ayurvedic practice has attracted what has seemed like an inordinate number of fertility patients, most in their late thirties or early forties. Clearly, in some cases infertility requires Western medical intervention. Ayurveda, however, addresses this issue from a truly holistic mind-body-spirit perspective.

The number of childless women has doubled since the 1970s. Between 1960 and 2015, the number of women giving birth has decreased by half. In a study of more than 8,800 women and 6,200 men between 2010 and 2012, 57 percent of women and 53 percent of men had a history of seeking help for infertility.

In the West, the first visit to a midwife or obstetrician takes place weeks after the pregnancy has been discovered, while in the East, the first visit to an Ayurvedic doctor typically takes place six months to a year before conception. It is understood that the health of mom and baby during and after pregnancy depends on the practice of time-tested Ayurvedic wisdom of pregnancy preparation and planning.

The first step of pregnancy planning and prep is the nesting process, where the mother and father prepare a safe environment in which to bring the new baby into the world. Studies support the ancient wisdom of pregnancy preparation, linking prenatal stress to issues related to maternal health, fetal health, and human development across the life span.

Unfortunately, as Heather so eloquently points out, we live in an extremely fast-paced, stressful time, and women in particular have been forced to live up to superwoman standards. While being a mom was once a full-time job, many women today must be not only the mom but also the chauffeur, soccer fan, cook, school liaison, social coordinator, travel planner, and often caregiver, all while holding down a pressure-ridden job. Now, they start out by trying to get pregnant, deliver, and care for an infant while already having a full plate of other responsibilities outside the home.

Trying to conceive in these conditions is about as impossible as a doe getting pregnant while being chased by a mountain lion. Getting pregnant requires a parasympathetic dominance in the nervous system that delivers a feeling of safety and security, according to Ayurveda. Stress has been argued to be a cause of infertility since ancient times, and today's studies back this up. In one study, 40 percent of women with infertility were shown to experience chronic high stress, anxiety, or depression prior to their first infertility clinic visit, suggesting that preconception stress may be an underlying factor of infertility.

Interestingly, in a study of six hundred female physicians, 24 percent of those who had attempted conception were diagnosed with infertility — nearly double the national average — another example linking prenatal stress with infertility.

Of course, this does not suggest that all infertility is due to chronic stress, depression, or anxiety. In fact, not all studies conclusively link prenatal stress to infertility, although there is overwhelming evidence that once a woman is diagnosed with infertility, her levels of stress, anxiety, and depression all go up, further complicating fertility. Counseling to reduce infertility-related stress and anxiety has been shown in a handful of studies to successfully boost pregnancy rates.

Pregnancy preparation is not a simple matter of changing a work or travel schedule; it is a process of slowing down in all areas of mom's and dad's life. According to Ayurveda, the dad's job is to fulfill the desires of the mom, including those wild cravings at 2 AM. The dad is also in charge of ensuring the mother's comfort, happiness, and joy by creating a calm, safe, peaceful environment, called *sattva* in Ayurveda. Peaceful, sattvic, supportive actions, such as touch, kindness, and caregiving between adults, have been shown to boost oxytocin, a birthing, bonding, and longevity hormone.

According to Ayurveda, pregnancy and delivery can be the most rejuvenating experiences of a woman's life, during which every cell of her body can be transformed. Traditionally, new mothers did not leave their bed for a week after delivery and did not leave the bedroom for two weeks, as the extended family provided meals, baths, and massages for mom and baby. Unfortunately, in the West, we did not get that memo, and mothers often pay dearly after pregnancy with further exhaustion, added stress, and other health concerns.

During pregnancy, downward-moving energy called *apana vata* supports development of the fetus, and upward-moving energy called *prana vata* supports mom's sattva, energy, and mood stability. In cases of chronic stress, both prana and apana can become depleted, leaving mom less able to cope with stress. In the battle for energy during pregnancy, the baby always wins, drawing both prana and apana to the fetus and leaving mom even more vulnerable to stress.

During the preconception period, these two energies must be restored in both mom and dad in the process of creating sattva in both parents. Depleted prana (mental energy) and apana (adrenal energy) not only impact the mom's chances to conceive, but can also deplete the quality and quantity of dad's sperm. Many studies link lack of sattva (aka a stressful lifestyle) to decreased fertility in men.

Rasayana for Pregnancy

To properly prepare for pregnancy and build sattva, future moms and dads have for thousands of years turned toward a branch of Ayurveda called *rasayana*, the study of rejuvenation, aging, and longevity. There are four main types of rasayana used traditionally to boost sattva and prepregnancy rejuvenation:

1. **Ahara rasayana** pertains to food and digestion
2. **Vihara rasayana** pertains to lifestyle
3. **Acharya rasayana** pertains to behavior
4. **Aushadha rasayana** pertains to herbs

These four types of rasayana focus on bringing sattva into the food, lifestyle, behavior, and herbs you consume. Sattva for pregnancy suggests that mom and dad be content, loving, kind, generous, grateful, compassionate, and joyful prior to conception.

Ahara Rasayana

Prior to conception, Ayurveda suggests bringing the body into balance. This starts with a thorough evaluation of the digestive system, followed by appropriate therapies to restore ideal digestive function. According to Ayurveda, the ability to digest well is linked to the ability to detoxify well and support a healthy immune response. During pregnancy, mom is doing all this for two — so baby's health starts with the digestive health of mom.

Vihara Rasayana

At least three months prior to conception is the best period for both mom and dad to cleanse physically, to rid the body of environmental pollutants and toxins as well as to emotionally shed *ama* (old, unwanted molecules of emotion) from mind and body.

Regular practice of gentle yoga, breathing exercises, meditation, walks in nature (thirty minutes each day), and breathing clean air are classic prepregnancy tools.

Daily full-body or foot massage with Ayurvedic oils will calm the nervous system and support a sattvic physiology.

Acharya Rasayana

Prior to conception, women are encouraged to read uplifting books and be with loved ones, engaging in uplifting conversation, as much as possible, rather than being alone.

Classic behavioral rasayanas also include the practices of truthfulness, devotion to love and compassion, nonviolence, living a pure and simple life, being free from anger and conceit, and being calm, sweet-spoken, positive, and respectful to elders and teachers.

Aushadha Rasayana

Ayurvedic herbal rasayanas are suggested to be taken for three to six months prior to pregnancy. Three classic preconception herbal rasayanas are chyawanprash, shatavari, and ashwagandha. These herbs have been used for thousands of years to support preparation for pregnancy.

The Ayurvedic Guide to Fertility is long overdue, and I am honored to write this foreword as this subject is very personal for me. My wife and I have raised six beautiful children using the principles of Ayurveda, and I am so grateful to Heather for writing this book so that many more can have access to this wisdom.

— Dr. John Douillard

Dr. John Douillard, DC, CAP, *is the creator of LifeSpa.com, the leading Ayurvedic health and wellness resource on the web, with over nine million views on YouTube and over 130,000 newsletter subscribers. Dr. John is the* *former Director of Player Development for the New Jersey Nets NBA team and the author of seven health books, including the Amazon bestsellers* Eat Wheat *and* The 3-Season Diet, *along with the newly released* Yoga Journal *video course* Ayurveda 201 *on Ayurvedic psychology. He is a repeat guest on the* Dr. Oz *show and currently directs LifeSpa Ayurvedic Clinic, the 2013 Holistic Wellness Center of the Year, in Boulder, Colorado.*

Introduction

How This Book Came About

Creativity — like human life itself — begins in darkness.
— JULIA CAMERON, *The Artist's Way*

The writing of this book arose of my own necessity to stay sane during a time of great uncertainty. I started writing parts of it years before I got pregnant as a sort of journal of things I was learning about how to preserve my fertility. I would save each page and file it away in a folder on my computer somewhere. It never occurred to me that I would be sharing my writing on fertility with anyone — until one day, after giving birth to my son, I decided to go back into the folder where I had tucked away every word.

What had I been writing about? I asked myself.

As I read through the titles of my writing, the themes began to emerge: the difficulty of deciding whether to have a child, the conflict between career and family planning, the concern about health issues that could potentially impede fertility, the fear resulting from not knowing if one can get pregnant, the benefits and risks of waiting until one is older, and the reality of only being able to control so much in the process. These were not only my issues. I also heard them come up over and over with my clients, colleagues, and friends. I knew there was something bigger than me that had to be addressed.

As a modern woman, I had always felt lucky to have the educational and career opportunities that women before me did not have, and at the same time, despite how great I considered my life to be, and even how good I considered my sex life, I always felt disconnected from my fertility. Not all of me was thriving in this new world. Once I hit my late thirties, I started to feel like my fertility was slipping away from me because I hadn't yet settled down with someone and didn't feel like my life was where I wanted it to be if I was going to become a mother. I did what a lot of women do today — I considered all my options as the clock was running out. I ran my hormones, contemplated egg freezing, and went on the hunt for a suitable partner. However, soon I realized that everything I was doing was based on the fear that I could not just make pregnancy happen.

It seemed to make sense that I would have approached fertility the same way I made everything else in my intellectual, professional, and physical life happen — with my thoughts, will, and efforts — except conception doesn't work that way. It requires far more receptivity and surrender. I made the vow that I was going to become a mother only if my body was ready for it and if the larger conditions of my life were favorable to it. And then, despite my fears about the biological clock, I stopped looking for ways to get pregnant and instead started tapping back into my primal nature. Going primal meant getting to know my body beyond the muscles, bones, skin, and fat. I had to get to know its history, emotions, desires, and urges. It also meant getting to know my menstrual cycles more.

When I decided to go primal, I wished there were a manual to tell me all the best-kept secrets of fertility that I could simply follow like a recipe and ease my mind. I looked through every ancient Ayurvedic medical text from India that I could find a decent English translation of and tried to locate this recipe. I tried to find it in the ancient yoga texts, too, then in the *Kama-sutra*, and in the great religious books that I had avoided for most of my life, but the recipe didn't exist in those places, either.

What I did learn from studying and practicing Ayurveda is that any symptom or event is merely the evidence of the mechanism behind it and that we have to go deeper to get at the actual patterns that created it. I knew that my own conception would happen only through focusing on the patterns of my life and health that would either support or hinder it. I spent two years working with one of the great women's health practitioners of the worldwide Ayurvedic community, Dr. Sarita Shrestha.

Since Dr. Shrestha lived in Nepal, I didn't get to meet with her very often — only once a year. Therefore, I spent most of my time trying to understand the principles behind her treatment advice and elaborate herbal formulas while studying my own body in my daily life. I began to understand my own emotions and how my body responded to the world around me. I uncovered attachments to things that were actually impeding how it functioned. I found deep-seated fear that I covered up with smarts and strength and control. I unearthed the wounds and the joys of my past. I found myself becoming so angry and sad at times that I wanted to punch the sky. These things were always there, but I had ignored them. Dr. Shrestha's guidance led me deeper inside myself. The study and practice of Ayurveda helped me understand what I was seeing so that I could detox, rejuvenate, and move forward into my future. Then, the universe started conspiring to make me a mother.

Your Fertility Journey

I've often wondered what determines whether a woman will become a mother. Obviously there are physical factors — like the condition of the body due to circumstances of birth, behavior, and environment — and there are mental factors having to do with confidence, vulnerability, and sexual and emotional intimacy. We might also suspect there is a third dimension completely outside of our control, the spiritual element. Is it simply written in the stars when we are born, or do we have any control over it whatsoever? Must we become obsessed to make it happen? Likely, the truth is somewhere in the middle of all this.

I've worked with women who wanted kids and didn't have them, and I've worked with those who didn't want them but had them anyway. It turns out that what we want isn't nearly as important as what happens. That is a difficult pill for a woman with a biological clock to swallow. However, it's not as if you should just say it's all out of your control. So much is within your power. This is the inspiration for this book: focus on what you can control, and leave the rest up to nature.

If you've picked up this book because you are considering becoming a mother, then welcome to the most insane ride of your life. Thankfully, there are billions of women who have been in your shoes before. Someone, somewhere, will understand your story.

If there are fears, blockages, or conflicts holding you back from having a child — well, it's time to face them. Not having children will not make these things go away. If you do not face them, they will remain and simply take on a new guise, in the form of wondering if you made the right decision once you hit perimenopause, and they will likely show up in other areas of your life, too. It's good to get your feelings about motherhood sorted out as early as possible, preferably while you are young, because the longer you wait, the more difficult the journey can become. Whatever you feel about motherhood now, it has nothing to do with how you will actually *be* as a mother. It has to do with your past. You really have no clue how you will be as a mother if you've never had a child.

Maybe you have already decided you want a child. This is wonderful, because now you can get started on your work. You are here to activate a channel that has been dormant or blocked for a long time. In doing this work, you will influence the course of your reproductive health, how you experience the world around you, and your overall life. The outcome is not clear, but that doesn't mean you shouldn't start the journey. At a minimum, you will learn far more about yourself than you've ever imagined.

How to Get the Most Out of the Book

In writing this book, I intend not so much to tell you how to become pregnant but rather to help you be your healthiest self on both an emotional and physical level *before* you become pregnant. I share tools and methods for you to achieve your best reproductive health through your day-to-day and seasonal practices — diet, lifestyle, sleep habits, work, and exercise routines, as well as yoga. By the end of this book, I want you to understand how you can best take care of yourself, and I hope that what you learn also helps you become a better mother, whatever you end up mothering in your life — whether it's a child, a furry little pet, or a passion project.

This book is here to inspire you and teach you about yourself and how your body works. We are going to cover some topics that are a little esoteric and spiritual and others that are very tangible and physical, like period blood and the excretions of your body. You are going to feel different dimensions of your being. We are also going to evaluate how you've been living your life. In some cases, you may feel a little confused from reading this book. That is a good sign.

You must prepare to ditch that which you are comfortable with. I want to show you how you've been limiting yourself. I want to show you how other people have been limiting you, too. I want to tell you that the grass is greener on the other side, but that the other side actually resides within you, not in another country, not with some other guy, not with some other job or that promotion, not with some medical test, and not even with the baby. The solution is right inside that sexy meat suit called *you*. Right now.

I haven't told you what I think is the worst part about this book: it offers no guarantee that you can have children even if you want them. It might not be in the cards for you. Just because you are reading this book doesn't mean you will definitely be able to have kids. It doesn't happen for everyone. The prize you are seeking isn't always the one you get at the end of your journey. However, there is always a prize, and in time only you will find out what that is. You simply have to keep putting one foot in front of the other.

If you are longing for a guarantee of what will happen at the end of this journey or for a shiny little pill you can take and magically have everything you want, then you will need to sit with that discomfort. I've been there myself, and I can tell you that some discomfort is always a part of a true spiritual journey.

And now, we take the next step.

Chapter 1

Fertility Today

Do not kill the instinct of the body for the glory of the pose.
— VANDA SCARAVELLI, *Awakening the Spine*

Becoming a mother is the ultimate yoga practice. My sisters, we are the torchbearers of one of the freakiest and most wonderful experiences a human can have — opening up and sharing the inside space of our bodies with another person and directly sharing a bloodstream, cells, energy, and nourishment. The problem is: we've gotten so good at *not* getting pregnant for most of our lives that we have all sorts of issues when we actually *want* to get pregnant!

When a woman wants to have a child — whether it's now or in the future — oftentimes a little thought crosses her mind: *When is the right time for me to get pregnant?* And if a woman has actually tried to get pregnant and is having difficulty, this thought shifts to: *Why can't I get pregnant? How can I get pregnant?* Women these days seem to have a lot of fear and insecurity around conception, as evidenced by the increase in measures taken by women today to try to control the outcome. Women are confused about what is best for their fertility and are grasping for help.

Even big corporate employers these days have picked up on this collective fertility insecurity. Many of the most competitive companies are now offering egg-freezing benefits to women in the workplace — women who dedicate their time, energy, love, and attention during the most fertile years of their lives to their jobs, rather than to starting a family.

But, over history, many women have had children and never planned it. They never thought much about how it would interfere with their lives, how they would continue building their careers or maintain a deep connection with their partners. They just had sex and rolled the dice. However, women today don't do anything by rolling the dice. Do we?

Modern women want to make sure everything is right when we do it. We love to strive. We love to make progress. We get a good degree, a good job, and a good performance review at work. When it comes to preparing for conception, we make no exception. We want to know if we're fertile ahead of time. We go get our Pap smears, pee on ovulation strips, check our hormones, do yoga, undergo acupuncture treatments, and expect conception to happen immediately because we're doing everything the way we were told to do it.

At the same time, as I mentioned, now women are masters of not getting pregnant. We have innumerable birth-control options, and it's become a societal norm to use them. Then we start to wonder what it really takes to turn it all around.

The good news is that, with a little care and attention — and some sexy lingerie — odds are, you can probably have a baby if you want to. I want to help you improve your overall health and your chances for conception so that you will have a better pregnancy and more ease as a mother down the road. Modern life has helped get you here, and now Ayurveda can help you better care for your fertility going forward.

Failing Fertility 101

Women have fewer children today than their mothers did. Between 1960 and 2015, the average number of children a woman gave birth to was reduced by half. The number of childless women has doubled since the 1970s, and the average woman in the world had 2.5 children in 2015, as opposed to 5 in 1960. But today's fertility landscape looks very different based on where you come from, what your religion is, how much money you have, and how many levels of schooling you've been through. Ironically, the women who seem the most successful — those with the best jobs, making the most money — are the least successful at having babies. Instead, it seems that putting so much energy and time into a career can rob a woman of the energy and time, and perhaps even the desire, she needs for fertility and motherhood. In addition, the stress levels that many women experience working in demanding jobs can end up sabotaging their health, damaging bodily tissues, crushing their creative spirit, and decreasing their reproductive power.

The women who are the *most* tapped into their fertility are actually women in less developed, less stable countries. For example, women in global areas of conflict, like Iraq, Afghanistan, and Yemen, have more than twice the number of children as do women in the stable, developed countries like the United States, Canada, and the United Kingdom. Of all the religious affiliations, Muslim women are the most fertile, having 24 percent more children than the world average, while Buddhists are the least fertile, having 36 percent fewer children than the world average. Women with less money are great at making babies. Younger women are also very good at it, but they are increasingly giving up their prime fertile years and waiting until later in life to start a family, typically to pursue education, careers, or travel.

In summary, the women who look like their lives have the comfort and independence that so many women today are striving for somehow seem to be the ones who are failing in the fertility department, while those women with seemingly more challenging lives are popping out kids like champs.

So why is the modern woman having difficulty with fertility? There are many reasons, but here are some of the more common ones: First, there are particular time frames when women are more fertile, and because many are now heeding the call of nature much later in life, they are missing the peak fertility windows. Second, modern women build very rich lives outside of family life. They can put all their energy into their passions and simply neglect the passion of creating a family. Third, in their quest for achieving the perfect life, modern women have lost an appreciation for events that happen outside of their control — which are, unfortunately, the majority of natural biological processes occurring in the body and in nature. And this third reason may be due to the fourth reason: the environment can be so toxic for women that it affects their health and creates confusion about whom or what they can trust.

When it comes to fertility, many women are limiting themselves by the very thing that appears to give them power in other areas. Modern women appear empowered and strong because they are going after the great career, breaking molds, or shattering glass ceilings, but they may be lacking in the areas of love and family. I find that many women in my Ayurvedic practice aren't even creating the space in their lives to meet a compatible partner, let alone start a family. Some dislike their jobs, bosses, colleagues, workload, or traveling so much — but they can't stop prioritizing these things above all other facets of life, including family.

Many let this go on until they reach a point where they don't feel they'll be able to reproduce naturally because they waited too long to have a child, and due to this, they undergo many years and thousands of dollars' worth of medical procedures to have a baby. Women try to outsmart time with the help of their doctors. Egg freezing, intrauterine insemination (IUI), in vitro fertilization (IVF), and getting a sperm donor and/or donor eggs and embryos are examples of the procedures a woman will undergo in order to check motherhood off her to-do list. Such an approach ends up working for some, and ends up with unfortunate outcomes for others. Even with egg freezing, there is always the risk that the freezer breaks. And root causes affecting fertility do not get addressed by focusing only on fertility treatment, and they can remain or get even worse after the baby is born.

And it's not just women who are having problems with fertility. Male infertility is also on the rise. The times are changing for both women and men who want to start a family. It's become difficult and expensive for so many people to have a child. However, there is also good news: the overwhelming majority of women who have children still conceive naturally, so there is hope for any woman looking to do so.

The Misaligned Superwoman

Today, modern women are exhausted, confused, and burned-out. Why else would we be so into yoga? We love burning ourselves out. Apparently, vacation time has been on a steady decline since 2000. A study done by Project: Time Off found that more than half of American workers left unused vacation days in 2018. And those who do take vacations frequently work while on them. With so many of us working like dogs, it's no wonder we are suffering from stress, anxiety, digestive disorders, insomnia, substance abuse, and so forth. Really, people? Is this what we've decided is the American dream?

I've been guilty of it myself. I remember canceling a vacation once when my team at work was implementing a critical project and I felt guilty leaving during such a difficult time. Guess what happened right after I called off this vacation? I got sick twice in one month. Oh, the irony: I canceled a vacation when I needed it most. I must have thought that no one else could function without me, or perhaps I didn't want anyone to function without me. What an ego. Truth is, if you work with a good team, then the moment you are out of the environment, people will shift around and start picking up the slack. Unless you are a key employee (this is fewer people than you may think), you are always replaceable, regardless of how late you work or how much time you put into that presentation.

Guess what happened when I left that job a year later? The work went on without me, as I went on my way with my work.

What have you done to burn yourself out in the past? What are you doing now?

A high percentage of people who experience stress (73 percent) report common psychological issues, such as irritability and anger, nervousness, lack of energy, or the urge to cry. An even higher percentage of people (77 percent) experience the common physical symptoms of stress, including fatigue, headache, upset stomach, muscle tension, and even loss of sex drive. So many of us are truly misaligned today. The wisdom of the body must be recaptured.

How we fill our free time is up to each of us. Some women will not take any time to relax or play, finding more and more opportunities to work themselves into the ground. Others are so lazy or so tired from work that they will sit in front of the TV all day or night.

It is important to look at yourself if either boredom or burnout is happening. They are two ends of the same spectrum. Either way, the wisdom of the body is being overridden by all the things you think you are supposed to be doing.

And this I can guarantee: However you are now, it's going to get magnified if you have a baby. Every pattern you have presently will become exaggerated if you give birth to a child and don't change your lifestyle because, in addition to having the same job, house payment, car payment, and so on, you will also have much more chaos and a tiny human depending on you who requires all the free time your sleep-deprived self can give.

What happened to listening to Mother Nature? Instead of being the intuitive goddesses women have been known to be throughout the ages, we are tiring ourselves out too much to truly listen. I can tell you where Mother Nature is: she's inside your body, and she's calling you home.

I've often wondered why we have so many yoga teachers today, myself included, and why the vast majority of yoga practitioners and teachers are women (which, oddly, is the complete opposite of how it is in India, where yoga was developed). Women are lost and confused. We are looking for more meaning. Things have gotten so crazy for us that we all need to go lie on the floor a couple of times a week and have some soothing voice tell us that everything is going to be okay, as long as we look within — and yet we don't truly look within and have to keep going to yoga class every week for a little break from life. This is not true healing. This is only a brief respite from the root causes. The world needs women to do yoga off their mats and go make themselves and the world a better place.

Undoing the Decades of Neglect

Modern culture doesn't celebrate feminine creative power very well. It celebrates women achieving things — becoming the CEO, starting the company, and doing it all with four kids. However, women are not taught much about the deep wisdom of their bodies and how to read it. I certainly was not.

If you had a woman in your life who thoroughly explained to you when you were a teenager what a treasure your body was, then consider yourself lucky. Many women today are educated about the female reproductive system in school, and only briefly. I still remember the day in fifth grade when the boys were taken outside to play kickball, and an educator proceeded to inform all us girls about the impending changes that would be happening to our bodies over the next few years. No one asked questions. We were all way too embarrassed. Here was an opportunity to teach us about the magical, mystical power we hold inside, and instead we felt traumatized. Like it or not, puberty was happening.

We are taught at this young age that we start to become different from boys, and that our bodies are something to be protected — from boys, from creepy adults, from pregnancy and sexually transmitted diseases. There is very little celebration of this newfound power awaiting us, and as a result, many of us do not learn how to fully tap into it and there's always an element of fear or disconnection surrounding our relationship with it. This often changes for us once we contemplate having a child. Suddenly we become very interested in this feature of our bodies that we felt was a nuisance for most our lives.

Biologically speaking, a woman develops the drive and capability to procreate at an age that is too young for her mind, family, religion, or culture to deal with. A young woman can have a baby once she goes through menarche (first period), which typically occurs between ages 10 and 15, with 12.6 being the mean age. Mentally and culturally, though, a budding woman at these ages is still developmentally a child. She has not yet matured enough to gain the level of independence or experience with the way of the world that an adult woman has. She is legally still a minor. Therefore, it is not socially acceptable for her to utilize this part of herself at the time it becomes biologically activated and available for use in the world, despite whatever normal, natural urges she has. If she is a responsible girl with urges, then in today's society, she immediately gets set on a course for blocking pregnancy that can last for decades.

As adult women, we are often confused by, and don't appreciate, our reproductive systems. We think they are way too inconvenient, and for years we mess with birth-control pills and other drugs to try not to have a period. If you are like me and lots of other modern women, then you spent most of your life using some form of birth control to avoid pregnancy. Perhaps you were so set on having sex whenever you wanted without getting pregnant that you even inserted a scratchy little IUD into your cervix to block sperm from getting in, even if it caused inflammation or hormonal imbalances. Maybe you wore a patch or even had some little implant placed. You let your intellectual and primal selves try to work together to solve the perennial problem of unplanned pregnancy until you felt ready for a planned one. You elicited help from your doctor to make this happen. And, when you finally decided that you might be ready for pregnancy, you began to feel that you had work to undo — to remove toxicity and blockages in both the mind and the body.

Most of my life, I wished I never had a period. It was a nuisance — something that got in the way when I wanted to go on vacation, work out, or have sex. I even went so far as to take the birth-control pill continuously for stretches of time so that I would never get a period. This was actually recommended to me by a gynecologist, so back then, I assumed it must have been a good idea. It was all very convenient for the other areas of my life, but after learning more about how the body works, I realized how narrowly focused our thinking is to cut off such a vital part of being a woman just because we find it inconvenient. A woman's body is meant to flush itself regularly even if it isn't getting pregnant — and perhaps especially if it's not getting pregnant.

Many women remain confused about whether they want to have kids until right before they think their biological clock is about to stop ticking, when confusion turns into panic and fear of missing out, and they wonder if they can still freeze their eggs. And then what ensues is either a hurried hunt for the father of their child or a dramatic letting go of the idea altogether and burying themselves back into work so they can forget about it — until perimenopause hits and everything blows up again.

If you have been physically or mentally blocking your reproductive energy, it's time to start to get to know this part of yourself again. Your awareness is power. By reacquainting yourself with your reproductive system, you will discover how truly magical it is. You are already, without a doubt, much more extraordinary than you've ever given yourself credit for.

Shifting from being a woman who has been blocking pregnancy to one who welcomes fertility is a multilevel process. It involves your mind, body, and spirit, and it's not just about you. Your partner is greatly affected. Your dynamic with this person and others in your life is in a potential transition state. Since you mean business now, it's time to look at all of this.

There is so much you can learn by studying your body, mind, cycles, and the environment around you. All your senses and several major systems of your body are involved in the monthly cycle, and if you are not paying attention to these cycles, you are missing out on some serious intuitive power — but when you reconnect with your inner being, even after trying to avoid pregnancy for so long, you are more likely to be reconnected with your reproductive power. When you turn a mirror back on yourself, you begin to see all the parts that may have been neglected or possibly even hurt. When you can see these clearly, then you can rejuvenate and heal and, in the process, develop superpowers.

Designing Your Life

Preparing your body for conception is really not that different from planting a garden. Once you learn what something needs to grow and thrive, you can create the conditions for that to occur: plant your seed during the right season, position it well, and then water accordingly. The first step is looking at what you yourself need in order to grow and thrive, and then you can focus on the elements that are supportive of building a family.

You must design a life moving toward bliss and health. To have these things, you need to cultivate the understanding that allows you to clearly perceive your environment. Then you have to make decisions that encompass your vision for your life, coupled with the reality in front of you. If you use your intellect wisely, you will make good decisions and health will prevail. If there is any flaw in your decision-making or in the use of your sense perception, then cycles of imbalances can begin.

It's really important that you be as healthy as possible before you conceive, because stuff gets crazy after you get pregnant and have a child. Just trust me on this. I hope you are excited about learning how to take really good care of yourself, because all your life experiences will be so much better if you have your best health, whether you have a kid or not.

Embracing the Unknown

The process of creation is not one that can be controlled — there are so many unknowns — and this can be a little unsettling for a lot of women. However, creation emerges out of vulnerability and even darkness. Creation is dominated by unseen forces that later give rise to something tangible and seen.

If you are considering having a child and you want the experience to be as joyous as possible, then first you must understand the process of how things are created and surrender to it. Creation comes from the need for change. It doesn't come when things are in perfect order. Otherwise, you wouldn't need anything different to happen in your life; there would be no space for something new.

There are variations on how conception occurs. Some women surrender to this process easily, and some after a glass of wine. Some women need to have doctors do it for them. Even when a woman goes to see a doctor for IVF or egg freezing or any other type of intervention used for conception, there is a form of surrender. It is just a different kind of surrender than getting pregnant the old-fashioned way.

Your job is to start to get comfortable in the darkness of space — when you don't have the answers or conclusions. Furthermore, your job as the female is specifically to let creativity happen *through* you. Yup, it's time to give up some of that control.

How do I sell this idea to you, though, if you are like a lot of other modern women and like to make vision boards and execute plans to get toward where you want to go? It can feel like a real struggle when we cannot make something happen via our own thinking and doing, can't it? It may feel difficult to let things unfold naturally until we feel we've done all we can. However, because conception takes more than one entity, a state of receptivity is important, and this can become compromised if we are trying to control everything. I'm not saying this is easy — receptivity and surrender challenge our fears around trust and even our own self-confidence.

In having a baby, you are not the one "making" anything when it actually happens. You are a vessel. You cannot control the outcome. You can try to influence it, but you can't control it. This is part of why a fertility journey — like any creative endeavor — is a spiritual journey for the modern woman who has a hard time relinquishing control. First, you do the best you can to take care of yourself in your environment, you connect deeply with your partner (literally and figuratively!), and then you roll the dice. You may experience mental anguish in the void, and this is where it's handy to hold a sense of faith and wonder. Allowing yourself to be surprised by the universe can actually be a really magical thing, sometimes even more fun than planning everything to a T and getting exactly what you want when you want it. Remember the saying "A watched pot never boils"? Well, it applies when you are trying to get pregnant, too.

Women who feel the call to conceive often start to grasp for a baby. They want to reach out and grab it, and they will do whatever they can to get it. Sometimes this works, and sometimes it sabotages the whole thing — because if there is too much grasping for the outcome, then there is no room for receiving the gifts that *take* you to the outcome. The baby you were meant to have will not come by your forcing. It will come by magic.

Pathologies are created energetically and physically when there are imbalances of giving, receiving, and grasping. Conception becomes blocked, elusive, or rejected when such pathologies are present. The balance point between receiving and giving is where you find the fertile ground for conception to take place.

How You Treat Your Body Matters

Physically, issues of under- or overnourishment of certain reproductive tissues will interfere with conception, so your diet and metabolism affect fertility. Some women are so undernourished that they don't have any energy for their menstrual cycle, and others are so overnourished (or wrongly nourished) that toxins and blockages begin to interfere with their normal metabolic processes, throwing off hormones and monthly cycles. Therefore, it is extremely important to get your diet and lifestyle equalized prior to trying to have a child. Some women benefit from cleansing and fasting to remove toxins and blockages, while others need more rejuvenation. Everyone, though, benefits by understanding their body type.

You want to take very good care of your body, internally and externally, especially if you wait until you are on the older end of the fertility spectrum. Older women generally pump out fewer follicles each month than younger women, and their bodies are often less moist and pliable. They typically do not get pregnant as easily and are more likely to have a C-section. You also need to take better care of your body if you've had any health issues that interfere with your general health or menstrual cycles.

Regardless of your age and health condition, having vigor and the ability to recover quickly is helpful, because being pregnant, giving birth, and nursing a small baby are all paradigm-shifting events for a body that can cause sleep deprivation, depletion, depression, and a whole host of not-so-fun things that you never hear about until you have a child. This is why it's important for you to focus on your own health *before* you get pregnant. It will make everything easier before, during, and after pregnancy.

Fertility through the Ages

Shortly after I had my own child at age thirty-nine, I was watching a group of young mothers on blankets at the beach with their little babies. They were energized, throwing their babies around, laughing, chatting, and smiling — all of them. Not one of the mothers looked the way I felt, which was completely zapped. I longingly mumbled under my breath, "They are so *young.*" I envied their energy and resilience. At the same time, when I heard the bubbly, twentysomething naivete of their conversations, I suddenly was happy I was bringing a child into the world with more years on me. There are pros and cons at every age. However, when it comes to fertility, the condition of the body is more important than what the mind says about anything, because the body always wins.

There are clear stages of biological life for a woman, beginning with infancy; going through childhood, puberty, adulthood, and perimenopause; and beyond menopause. The stages do not fall on exactly the same years for all women, because women have different birth constitutions and age at different rates for various reasons, but the general pathway is the same. The first part of life is a time for building the body, the middle is for maintenance, and the body breaks down more in the final phase of life.

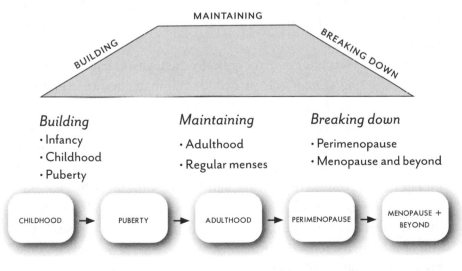

Figure 1: The life stages of a woman

There are different strengths, weaknesses, and vulnerabilities in each of life's phases. When it comes to deciding when to have a child, every woman has to find her own sweet spot based on her own constitution, how she lives her life, her intimate relationships, and the sort of support she has around her, although I would argue that the current trend of women having children later and later may be socially and financially beneficial but generally is not biologically beneficial. The body is more resilient when it is younger, which is very handy when having a kid because gestating, birthing, breastfeeding, and lugging around a toddler can be seriously physically challenging athletic endeavors. It's also easier to deal with sleep deprivation when you are younger, and new parents inevitably become wickedly sleep challenged for a few months and even a few years.

It All Starts in the Teenage Years

When we look at a child or even a teenager, it can feel a little weird to think of that individual as a sexual creature, but the reality is that most girls and boys hit puberty when they are still children — many even before they are teenagers. Not only that, but most females become sexually active in their teenage years. Only 17 percent of women are still virgins into their nineteenth year. Assuming you are an adult woman now, the defining relationship with your reproductive system started a very long time ago.

The early years after puberty, typically the teens, are not an optimal time for a young woman to have a child. A woman's body is still developing, essentially practicing its menstrual cycles and continuing its way through the awkward years following onset of puberty. Add to this any moral considerations, plus the fact that she is still legally a minor until she is eighteen and is typically financially and socially dependent on her parents during these years, and it makes it especially challenging for a teenage girl to deal with her own sex drive and developing intimate relationships when, inside, so much is changing for her. At the end of the day, if a female is ovulating, then she could possibly become pregnant, so this is indeed a tricky time of life!

The teenager of the modern society is more than likely going to

wait until her twenties, thirties, or forties before she has a child. However, the teenage years are an important time, because how she handles
her sexual urge and manages her menstrual cycle and reproductive
functioning in this stage of life will influence her sexuality and overall
health for years to come.

In these next sections, we'll break down the phases of the fertile
era — from young women to mature women, terms used loosely because women are aging at different rates due to differences in constitution, lifestyle, and environmental factors.

Young, Fertile Women

A healthy twentysomething's body is robust and juicy. She is in her
physical prime, an ideal time to have a child. Her body is already mature enough to conceive, gestate, birth, and breastfeed a baby. Children
are very juicy, and a young woman carries this juiciness with her into
her womanhood. A woman's ability to heal and rejuvenate after a physical trauma (which is often what giving birth is!) is typically stronger
at this time of life.

The earth and water elements are plentiful when women are young,
and these become magnified as the fire element starts to increase in
puberty. The increasing fire element gives a woman greater intensity
and influence over her environment. She has only to choose where this
energy goes.

Young women are increasingly delaying having children until they
are in their thirties and even their forties. As of 2012, less than 50 percent of women had a child by the end of their twenties, and these numbers are still decreasing today. Many women are placing the rest of life
in front of having a child, especially if they are educated. These women
are also delaying marriage more and more. Many women have a feeling
that there are things they want to do before they become a mother.
This creates a paradox for a young woman because while her body
may be completely ready to have a child, her mind and oftentimes her
support network are not. Depending on her culture and specific life
history, she may not feel ready to have a child yet. However, if she does
have a child, then she's doing it at the generally best time biologically.

Despite increasingly not wanting to have kids until later, young women are often sexually active and using some form of birth control. In my practice in the San Francisco Bay Area, where I've worked with hundreds of people, I have had only one twentysomething client who was abstinent by choice, and she did so for religious and spiritual reasons. But regardless of her reason, I observed that she was one of the most aligned individuals I'd come across in my years working with clients. She knew she didn't want to get pregnant — and so she just didn't have sex. She was old enough. She was mature enough. She was even living with her fiancé. However, she planned to remain abstinent until they got married. I remember thinking: *Wow, that must be hard to do!* In a sexually liberal city like San Francisco, you don't meet many people who are abstinent by choice! I noticed she was also very diligent about her eating and exercise routines — apparently not having sex gives you energy for lots of other things. Or perhaps she just had more self-control than most people.

A young woman is not in a rush to be a mother nowadays, because she believes she has many more years ahead of her to get pregnant and have a family, especially after seeing so many older women have children. The clock does not tick for her — except when it comes to her fears about the future. Young women still experience fear of missing out on having kids when they direct their energy elsewhere, and more of them are resorting to egg freezing. Given that the big companies that a lot of these women work for are increasingly offering their female employers egg freezing as a health benefit, it's clear that young women are still concerned about waiting to become mothers. Freezing their eggs feels like an insurance policy in case they end up waiting too long to get pregnant. However, an older woman with frozen eggs will still be left with her own older body, which will need to be medically assisted in the process of becoming pregnant. It's not just the eggs that matter; the rest of a woman's body matters, too, and the seasons of life can be manipulated only so far. We can outsmart nature only so much, and there are usually consequences when we do.

But where do the thirtysomethings fall? This is the decade in which a woman often feels the most pressure about having kids (unless she's still in limbo into her forties, of course!). It is also, coincidentally, the decade in which many women seem to have some sort of midlife crisis — myself included. The thirties can be an empowering decade for a woman, but they can also be confusing if she has gotten out of alignment in some way — physically, mentally, or spiritually.

Thirtysomethings go in one of two camps — early thirtysomethings can oftentimes put themselves in the "young woman" category if they still feel physically young, but as forty looms, those who have read the data on fertility and listened to what everyone else around them says about it will likely start to put themselves in the "mature woman" box. The midlife crisis so many women experience in this decade has to do with how they're living their overall lives, and oftentimes, fertility is a major factor. Some women go through this crisis before having their kids, and some have it afterward. I had mine beforehand.

Some women in their thirties are worrying about their fertility for good reason, and other women are worrying about it for no reason at all, but it doesn't have to do with age so much as it does with how a woman cares for herself and what sort of environment she is in. Doctors typically say that a woman conceiving at thirty-five or over is a high-risk pregnancy, and it can be a little unsettling when you feel absolutely fine and your doctor tells you that you are a *geriatric* pregnant patient (the actual term used for pregnant women over thirty-five). The problem is that once someone throws a number out as a guideline, saying it's the average age when something happens, then people stop seeing possibilities and start looking only at numbers.

The reason this is sad is because everyone is aging at different rates. Time matters, but only insofar as it is relevant to the individual's constitution, lifestyle, and environment. Some women are actually aging faster, and some are aging more slowly. Women do not all first get their periods at the same age, do they? And we all start menopause at different ages, too. Therefore, our fertile windows can also be different.

A woman is much better off studying her own body — the quality of the tissues; her ability to heal and regenerate; the quality of her hair, skin, nails, sleep, digestion, and menstrual cycles; and how she feels emotionally — to analyze basic physiological functions and features. She may just be a little bit different from her peers and even from her family members. She may have more years left than she thought, or she may have already missed her chance. The key is for her to pay attention to her body.

Mature, Fertile Women

Once you hit thirty, thirty-five, forty, or whatever age you consider yourself a more mature woman, it's good to forget about the numbers for a moment and take a very objective look at your body. The later chapters in this book will help you evaluate it, but I will give you a hint now that the key is in the five elements: *space, air, fire, water,* and *earth.*

As our fire increases at puberty and builds into middle age, it eventually burns away some of our earth and water. The question is not *if* this will happen but *when.* With healthy aging, we become a little less like a watery, chubby baby and more like a shaped and refined piece of fine pottery. However, if the earth and water elements get a little too depleted, then we burn out and dry out, increasing the air and space elements and moving toward breakdown, degeneration, and even inflammatory issues.

Women who have a well-functioning, juicy body and manage their health well in their youth may be in better shape to have a child during their mature years, just as women who have signs of early aging and degeneration may not have as long a fertile window, because the air element has already begun to take over. A mature woman feels a greater disruption to her overall lifestyle when she has children because she's lived her old life longer and is used to it. Therefore, the new state feels like a big psychological and behavioral shift. In addition, the more mature body needs more time to rest and rejuvenate after going through such a significant physical and emotional event, but she can manage that by building support around her.

It is always best to get an honest and raw understanding of the condition of your one-of-a-kind body using the senses. What do you see, taste, smell, hear, and feel? What is underneath the makeup or the hair dye? What happens when you don't wear deodorant? What kind of condition is your skin really in? How about the teeth and the gums? Sometimes the small things you might want to fix cosmetically are telling you something critical about your health. One tissue can become affected by an imbalance more than others. The key is to pay attention and know yourself for how you really are.

Let's say you find that you aren't really showing many signs of aging or toxicity — both issues for fertility. For example, your skin still seems juicy and thick. Your hair is still lustrous and is mostly not gray. You still get regular, effective periods, and the flow patterns seem relatively unchanged. Your injuries heal fairly easily. You have an appetite. You don't have any cysts or other growths. You generally sleep well at night. These are just a few examples of youthful health. If you consider yourself a mature woman and yet your body still maintains a healthy quality and vitality, then you might be one of the lucky women in their older fertile years who may do just fine having a kid.

If you are feeling like the clock might be ticking, then still, it's not time to freak out; it's simply time to truly look at your body and position yourself for the best health possible (again, something I hope to help you with in this book).

I've had women in their early forties start working with me thinking that they are going through early perimenopause, and in all cases they were wrong — they were just going through a life transition that was interrupting the basic physiological processes involved in menstruation and throwing off the rest of their health, too. It's not that early menopause doesn't happen to some women — it's just very rare. It happens in about 5 percent of women.

If you feel healthy and strong and like you still have your youthful glow and juiciness, then you may be in good condition to have children for years to come. If you feel like you may need to improve your health, then this book will help you reclaim your vitality. Regardless of your age, take care of yourself, and if you do end up having a kid, I would suggest that you devote your energy to lining up support around you to help with postpartum rejuvenation and childcare — even if you are a stay-at-home mom. The transition from nonmother to mother can be challenging for many women — even if they desperately craved a baby — but it's worth it.

Chapter 2

Going Primal

Let your mind go, and your body will follow.
— HARRIS K. TELEMACHER, played by Steve Martin, *L.A. Story*

I have some news for you. Wanting a baby is not what creates a baby. Thinking about a baby doesn't create a baby. It is your physical desire to have sex with your male partner when you are fertile, plus his reciprocated desire and the two of you acting upon it, that will get you pregnant. I actually believe that wanting a baby too strongly gets in the way of natural conception because it focuses energy and attention ever so subtly away from the actual act needed to make the baby.

The process of creation is an animalistic act that allows for a mystical event to occur, and this produces real, physical results…a new person! It is unmistakably a spiritual process — in the sense that it's beyond material understanding. There are fundamental parts of it that cannot be grasped by the mind or by modern science. No one understands how a soul enters a cell, or group of cells, and when this occurs. Similarly, no one knows when a soul leaves a body. There is always more going on than we can understand.

A student once asked the great yogi Paramahansa Yogananda, author of *Autobiography of a Yogi*, when the soul enters the body. He stated that it happens at the moment of conception; that there are essentially souls waiting for the moment of conception to occur so that they may enter. Waiting where? Yogis call it the astral world. It's supposedly beyond the physical world and the mind. Perhaps it's that place we tap into in dreams. Yogananda believed that upon conception, a spark of light is released in that astral world, and that's the cue for the soul to come on into the egg and sperm's newly formed arrangement of matter. Maybe this is also related to the light people say they see when they are near death. Perhaps that's not an ending but rather the beginning of something else.

And despite all religions and physicists attempting to define how creation occurs, ultimately, none of the best and brightest minds we know really understand it. This makes total sense, because creation is not a conscious, thinking process. Rather, it's a deep, dark, and mysterious one.

You don't need to meticulously think your way into creating a baby, but your thinking mind really does not like to hear this. Your thinking mind wants to feel like someone or something is within your control. The idea that events actually happen some other way, possibly even randomly, is a discomforting thought for you if you are like most modern women. We like predictability, control, and surety, and many of us find concepts like *faith*, *trust*, and *surrender* to be challenging. What exactly are we surrendering to?

Regardless of your religious or spiritual leaning, I hope we can agree that you have a body, a mind, senses, and a soul, and each of these dimensions plays a major role in every moment of your life, including conceiving a child. You know what your body is because you can see it. You have an idea what your mind is because you can hear it chattering all the time when life goes quiet. Your senses — hearing, feeling, seeing, tasting, and smelling — are used daily for basic life functions and experiencing pleasure and pain, so you have a tangible grasp of how they work. However, the soul is where the human animal gets a little more confusing.

In Sanskrit, the word *atman* is used to refer to soul or spirit. Yogis believe that the atman is beyond the physical body and the mind, and yet it permeates everything. Whatever you can observe, then, is atman, but you can't perceive it with your senses. This elusiveness would make it very difficult for a scientist to find the atman, because science needs to be able to observe something to prove that it's there. Atman is even *more* confusing because it is both very small and very big. The very fact that such opposites can exist simultaneously is precisely why the soul transcends the conscious mind. Just try making sense of it!

The main reason the atman is so ubiquitous is because it is the witness seeing everything, so a person cannot directly observe it. In order to observe it, one would have to turn the awareness back toward oneself and then not get distracted at all by thoughts, memories, or the body on the way there. But who doesn't get distracted by these things in today's world? We think all the time. We cling to the past. We fear the future — and we feel physical stress, pleasure, and pain, so the body is a highly distractible object.

In fact, this reversing of the awareness toward yourself to discover the soul has always been the goal of yoga practice, despite its modern reputation as a way to turn your body into a strong, flexible, or more slowly moving pretzel in order to reduce stress.

The word *yoga* also comes from Sanskrit, and it actually means "to yoke together." In yoga, we're in a state of complete connectedness with an object of focus, without distraction. In all other states that aren't yoga, distraction exists, as witnessed in the chattering of the mind that is present. In order for us to truly connect with anything, the noise must be silenced. We must achieve presence.

This search for soul is part of the yoga journey, whatever your version of yoga is. For example, right now, you are doing the yoga of book reading.

Cultivating Your Psychospiritual State

How many times have you heard of a woman who tried to get pregnant for a long time undergoing all sorts of invasive medical procedures for years; possibly beginning to search for alternative ways of baby making, such as surrogacy or egg donation; starting to look into adoption; or relinquishing the idea altogether — and then someday, when she's given up completely, she magically conceives a child? What a ride. When I see this, it always makes me wonder: *Was all this necessary? If she had done things differently, could she have still gotten to the same place?*

Your state of mind is important for this journey, as is your sense of connectedness with spirit. Remember, getting too narrowly focused on the goal of having a baby will not help you, because you will lose sight of what it takes to make a baby. If you are already stuck obsessing about this goal, it's time to explore the deep places inside you and ask bigger questions about the nature of life and the universe — so that you actually become open to new possibilities. Everything exists as possibility before it becomes reality.

Presence is also important for this journey. That means not being stuck in the past or thinking about the future. You might be lucky and unexpectedly get pregnant after a night of wining and dining on a hot date with the one you love. I say this is lucky, because the moment your mind becomes engaged in thinking about pregnancy, it can actually end up getting in the way, because it distracts from presence. Once you start planning, analyzing, scenario building, or scheming, this is often where the process becomes stressful and you have probably gotten off track from the cosmic, creative magic of it.

Natural pregnancy occurs in a way that is part predictable and part mysterious. When you are in a place where things seem a bit like they don't make sense, you are probably on the right track. Having a sense of wonder is important. However, if you start trying to make everything happen the way you want it to, you may become frustrated. This would be a fruitless effort if you've never been pregnant before, because you really have no clue how it will happen, even if you are a healthcare practitioner or biomedical scientist and have lots of intellectual knowledge of biological reproduction.

Conception involves two people and the universe, and all three have to be on board for it to occur. Women have shared countless stories with me of undergoing painful medical procedures to become pregnant, and some without any luck for years. Imagine: chasing pregnancy as a goal, and it doesn't happen when you want it to — for years? The women I've worked with in this situation are angry, frustrated, and devastated. Not getting what you want can be so soul crushing that some women begin to question everything.

I myself had to drop to my knees and weep a few times in my journey. However, it was in these painful moments, too, that I discovered a type of magic. I'm telling you — this journey may look messy and frustrating at times, but it will also bring some unexpected gifts.

The Primal vs. Intellectual Self

The modern woman has two minds. If these two minds are not on the same page, then they can wreak havoc on her life, but when they are in harmony, they can create magic, poetry, and little people. The two minds are the intellectual and the primal. You could call them the conscious and the subconscious. One of the dimensions is conscious mental activity, intellect, and thought. This mind likes ideas, stories, and information. The other is subconscious, in charge of about 95 percent of the body's operations, with all its sensations, emotions, drives, and urges. These two minds coexist, but sometimes it feels like they are not in accord. Moreover, the dimension that you have less awareness of is the one running most of the show. Take a guess about which one you think will win if there is a conflict between the two.

You are both an intellectual and animal creature. Your intellect has the ability to understand what is good and bad, make decisions, strategize, and so forth. You can learn quickly in school, get the gold star for your homework, and later get that great internship or job. You can also make the decision to work late and overachieve, go to the gym, go home and cook dinner, or go on a date. All this is the job of your intellect.

Your primal self is ancient. It was passed down to you from generations long ago, and then it's been iterated based on your life experiences and choices. It's been influenced by your intellectual self. The primal wants to synchronize with the primordial rhythm of nature, and it does so whenever your choices and actions within an environment allow it to. However, the primal is also the space where emotions are felt, and if you are not used to listening to your emotions and letting them inform your decisions, then you will become misaligned and be unable to connect with the rhythm of nature.

You are smart but not perfect. You get hurt, and sometimes you even make mistakes. And you have blind spots. You are an emotional being — not a computer. This is what makes you human.

Women today need a pathway to explore their inner animals because our day-to-day lives are now spent in structures and systems that were originally designed by men, for men. And the wellness practices and teachings that many of us use to undo the effects of being caught up in this man's world — modern yoga practices, for instance, or mindfulness — remain mostly focused on the mind, muscles, and bones, which are the areas of thoughts, will, and structure. Women today need practices and teachings that bring them into the more rooted realm of the emotions and urges.

The word *buddha* means one who has achieved enlightenment, but a female buddha will figure out how to simultaneously listen to the deep and ancient, unconscious spaces in her body, learning how to read the psychophysical experiences of her emotions, and translate these into wise actions. Since the primal animal is such a huge part of a woman, the mindful woman gets to know it more closely — especially when she's contemplating having a baby. Getting pregnant, being pregnant, giving birth, and raising a child can be the most embodied experiences a female buddha can have in this modern life.

A woman who places too much value on her thoughts, ideas, will, and structure and does not balance that out with the exploration of her inner animal — her emotions, gut, heart, and reproductive functioning, including the 95 percent of her programming that isn't conscious — will experience mental stress and bodily imbalance. A stressed-out woman can spend years and years reprogramming her mind via all sorts of training or therapies, but if she does not get into the experience of her body, and the emotions experienced inside, then she cannot make the changes necessary to realign her life back with nature, and she will get caught in a never-ending battle between the two selves. If she doesn't learn to talk with her body, then that body will always seem to fail her.

So here's the question: Can you let go of what you know to be your mind, the intellectual part, and tap into your primal dimension?

I'm not insinuating that the mind is not important. It is just as important as the animal self. A state of health comes from making good decisions, and most of the maladies we face in life are the result of the intellect being misused somewhere along the way. For the modern woman, one of the greatest misuses is not getting to know her animal self better, and instead aligning with meaningless pursuits until she wakes up. If she gets to know the animal self deeply, then her intellect can actually arrive at better-informed decisions, which will make her life more efficient, her body healthier, and her spirit more alive.

Getting in touch with your reproductive power requires that you dive a little more into the dark, mystical realm where you don't already know everything and where it can be difficult to draw conclusions. You may feel confused. Things may not make sense. However, once you journey into this magical, primal space, you can clear a pathway for being receptive to the ultimate creative endeavor.

Going Deeper into Your Body

Once I was adjusting a yoga client as he held a pose for a long time, and he said to me, "Is it fucked up that I want things that are bad for me?" My heart sank. I felt his contrition, and at the same time, I knew I was guilty of this, too. Our minds oftentimes override a healthy, natural decision in favor of what we think we are *supposed* to do, and we've been trained to do this from a very young age.

It can be confusing to discern what is an urge of the body and what is an urge of the mind. The body sends feelings — sensations, emotions, and the like. The mind has thoughts. Your body feels something and then your mind tells you a story about it, and vice versa — when your mind tells you a story, your body feels something. Finding your truth can be difficult because sometimes your mind is confused or missing very important information.

It's time to tap into the wise lady that lives within you. You are very smart when you pay attention. You cannot fully tap into your intuition if you are distracted by your thoughts. Intuition is what happens spontaneously when you have connected the two minds.

To tap into this power, you must begin to observe both your thoughts and your bodily responses. If you listen closely, you will see how your body reacts in certain situations — sometimes unexpectedly — and can begin to try to understand these reactions. The body is great at telling us that we need to make a different decision: allergies, digestive issues, energy depletion, irregular periods, and sleep or skin problems are a few examples of this. However, sometimes you may not heed the body's call, and the solutions your mind comes up with when the body is experiencing discomfort are not so effective for relieving it.

An example is drinking more coffee or exercising a lot to get over your tiredness from either lack of sleep or not eating well for your constitutional type. When you don't resolve the root cause, it ultimately is the source of more stress and anxiety and sabotages sleep even further, which then creates the stronger dependence on caffeine. Then you realize that you are getting headaches when you don't have your caffeine, and the addiction persists. When you finally wake up and realize that such excessive amounts of caffeine are damaging your body, you have to go through withdrawal headaches, so then you have to take some sort of headache medicine in the process. What your mind prioritizes is sometimes not beneficial to your health or aligned with what you truly desire for your life.

To dive back into the primal, not only must a woman pay closer attention to her mind and body, but she must also learn to trust that the body knows what is best. The Ayurvedic approach to health requires that whenever there is a conflict between mind and body, the cues of the body win. The body is biological. The mind is fleeting.

Whenever you feel torn because of a battle between your head and your heart, it is really this battle between your thoughts and the sensations and emotions being felt in your body. Even while thinking, you will often find that your body sends you a signal. If you listen to your body's responses with a finely tuned ear, you will move toward a place of health. If you follow your thoughts without listening to your body, a healthy way of being may elude you.

Connecting Mind with Body

To connect the mind with the body, most people today need to learn how to sense the body more. You may be used to doing yoga, dance, or fitness exercises, which is a good way to develop a deeper connection with the body. Any study of one's movement, will, and actions is a worthwhile endeavor in understanding the self. There is, however, an additional dimension to connect with that can provide a good bridge between the mind and the body. This is the energetic layer, and the yogis throughout history have done a pretty good job trying to paint a picture of it.

The base of the spine is considered the seat of *kundalini* energy, known as primal serpent energy. This energy can be either dormant or awakened — the serpent coiled or rising — and if awakened, will travel upward and activate an individual at different levels and dimensions. This upward-moving energy is the crown jewel of those individuals looking to awaken their whole being, and it can occur for many reasons — either spontaneously or through guidance from a teacher. The *chakras* are the body's seven main energy centers, which are oriented along the spinal column, from the base of the spine to the crown of the head. When kundalini activates the chakras above the heart, much of the energy goes toward communication and thought, whereas the energy in the lower chakras is more primal, fueling digestion, sexuality, and excretion.

With so much emphasis on thought and intellectual activity in our day-to-day lives, many women today have too much going on in their upper chakras. The prevalence of head-forward body postures is largely due to this overuse of the mind, reflected in the habit of sitting in front of a computer or staring at a mobile device, reading, viewing, thinking, and achieving through thoughts and communication. However, a healthy person will have balanced energy throughout the body and will not be dominated by one chakra center or the other. What this means for a lot of us is that we need to let go of our overuse of the mind.

Focusing on any one of the chakras will redirect awareness and energy to that center. For example, focusing on the lowest chakras brings awareness to the pelvic basin, and focusing on the center of the chest brings awareness to love and the rhythm of the heart. Focusing on the center of the belly will connect you with your willpower, and focusing on the throat brings energy to the voice. When you notice that certain chakras feel blocked or overactive, which can happen when the mind, physical body, or emotions have gotten out of balance, you can focus on the other chakras to shift the energy, or you can choose to go deeper into a blocked chakra to understand its mental-emotional-physical components.

In addition to chakra exploration practices, there is a spot you can activate that will bring you back to your primal energy: a point at the base of the skull that yogis refer to as *mastaka granthi*, or "head knot." Mastaka granthi is located at the site of the brain stem, specifically the medulla oblongata. We know from modern science that the brain stem is the relay system between the brain and the rest of the body, and is also the control center for certain fundamental functions of the autonomic nervous system, or primal body, including consciousness, breathing, cardiovascular activity, and the natural, reflexive urges like sneezing and vomiting. It is a regulating center of a whole bunch of stuff that the intellect isn't necessarily involved in. Mastaka granthi is the gateway between the head and the body — a space between — where the intellectual dimension surrenders to the primal, biological, animal state of the body, and vice versa. This is a useful spot to know about because while it is great to journey on the path to motherhood with balanced chakras, it's even better to deeply get in touch with your basic biological functions.

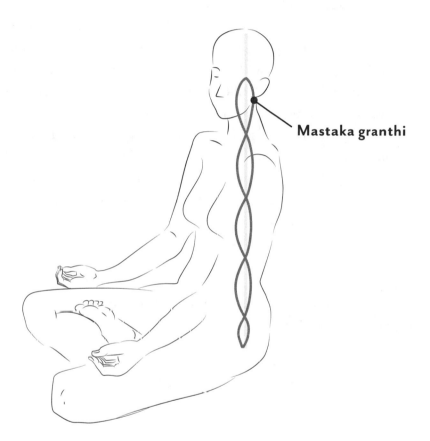

Mastaka granthi

Figure 2: Kundalini rising through the chakras, harmonized with mastaka granthi

Next, I offer a practice for you to walk through this primal doorway before we dive into some Ayurvedic health principles in the next chapter.

EXERCISE: MERGING THE PRIMAL AND THE INTELLECTUAL

As we begin this journey to align your mind, body, and spirit and improve your reproductive health, you can begin by connecting your mind with your body.

With a neutral, nontilted chin, take your left index and middle fingers and begin gently massaging high on the back of your neck. As you move your fingers around with very soft pressure, you may notice a small valley in the top center of your neck between the muscles on either side of the spine.

Keep slowly moving the left middle finger upward until you find a tiny cavern at the base of the skull. Once you have found that point, lightly rest the pad of your left middle finger in that little spot. You have found mastaka granthi. Continue to hold your finger there gently.

Chant *om* silently to yourself.

Walking through this doorway, you are beginning to align to the primal rhythm.

Chapter 3

Principles of Health

I believe it's really about unfolding ourselves.
— **ANGELA FARMER,** *The Feminine Unfolding*

Ayurveda *means "the science of life,"* and it is considered to be a sister science to the practice of yoga. I first discovered Ayurvedic medicine while studying to be a yoga therapist in my early thirties. I was taught just a smidgen of Ayurveda and became so fascinated that I entered a graduate program to study more. In India, it is a very old and well-established form of medicine, and today there are hundreds of thousands of Ayurvedic doctors and practitioners in India. Along with traditional Chinese medicine, which most people know by one of its popular therapies, acupuncture, Ayurveda is one of the oldest systems of medicine in the world. I had been practicing yoga and meditation for years, which helped me learn how to master my will and effort and influence my nervous system, but Ayurveda helped me unlock the golden door of understanding nature and how our cells, bodies, and minds are connected to the larger macrocosm.

In the United States, barely anyone had heard of Ayurvedic medicine when I was studying it, though it has gotten wildly popular in the last few years in the wellness world. Even now, you will see mixed feedback about it if you research it online. Some sources will say it's the great mother of all medicines, the most transformative form of healing ever to be found. Others will say it's quackery and practiced by snake-oil-salesman practitioners. Ayurveda is actually a medical philosophy that's been around for thousands of years, so it comes in many forms and is difficult to nail down. It's been referred to as ubiquitous, or present everywhere, because its principles have been applied in so many areas — from beauty products, foods, and medicines, all the way to self-help literature and the classes at your local yoga studio. For me, it just made complete sense the first moment I heard about it, and the more I learned about and practiced it, the better my health was and the more alive I felt.

I was more connected to nature. I noticed the moon in the sky more. The plants and trees were suddenly more interesting. And it finally gave me words, albeit in Sanskrit, to explain things I had felt for a long time but had no way to express. Before I knew it, I left my well-paying corporate career in the health-insurance industry to study a foreign form of medicine that no one I knew had heard of or could even pronounce.

Like traditional Chinese medicine, Ayurveda is based on a five-elements model of health, the five elements being space, air, fire, water, and earth. They provide an uncomplicated, intuitive way to describe what is happening in nature and in a body and its environment. The five elements can be used to understand the properties of what a body ingests, and how these properties show up in tissues and physiology during states of imbalance.

The body is a collection of channels through which air, energy, sound, and different substances and materials travel. Channels go in and out of cells, organs, and tissues. The integrity of the channels is paramount in Ayurvedic medicine. A healthy body has freely flowing channels, and when these channels are overwhelmed, blocked, or damaged, there is some imbalance in the body. Imbalances cause disease, and we don't want disease if we are trying to conceive. We want to be a receptive and resilient channel.

So how do we nip imbalances in the bud? Modern medicine typically isn't very effective unless there is some emergency going on. Even then, when the modern medical system solves a problem with drugs or surgical or device intervention, it often ends up creating another problem altogether. True healing is found in other places these days, and it all starts with you.

Healing now will make things easier for you down the road when you conceive. Studying your body can tell you a lot. Pain, inflammation, swelling, digestive issues, skin problems, headaches, tissue growths, and PMS symptoms signal that something needs to be looked at more closely, especially if the patterns remain persistent or get worse over time. Noticing quickly when the body is in a state of health versus a state of imbalance can make all the difference in trying to reverse disease processes. However, if you are like most people, you pay attention to your work, your friends and family, the news, or your thoughts more than you do your own body. That was me when I was in my thirties — until I realized that I'd been dragging this body around with me my whole life and knew very little about how it worked.

We aren't given a manual on how our bodies work when we are born. Even trained medical professionals don't always fully integrate their learning on the body, because intellectual knowledge, helping other people, and our own embodiment are completely different things. When I started studying my own body, I noticed how complex it was — how so much is going on all the time in all its nooks and crannies. I felt overwhelmed by how much there was to learn, and it seemed it would take forever to truly understand it. I wondered: *Is there a way to learn about health that is instead really simple and won't feel daunting to tackle?* Ayurveda was my answer.

Ayurveda gives insight into the very beginnings of disease by studying seemingly benign symptoms that most people simply discount because they can oftentimes take some over-the-counter medicine for them, but they are a big deal if they persist. All disease conditions — minor or major — have their roots in these small health issues. To prevent and reverse disease, you want to catch it as early as possible, because it's more and more difficult to address it as time goes on. The good news, which I will explain in subsequent chapters, is that imbalance follows very specific patterns, so if you pay attention, you will be able to detect and rebalance issues.

My goal is to introduce you to a few helpful concepts from Ayurvedic medicine so that you can discover how you can be your healthiest self. In introducing Ayurveda to you, I fear I will convey only a fraction of the brilliance of this medicine, because it is so very vast and wise. Nevertheless, I will try. In some cases I will use transliterated Sanskrit terms because there is no meaningful English equivalent to express certain concepts.

Definition of Health

A person with [a] uniformly healthy digestion, and whose bodily humours are in a state of equilibrium, and in whom the fundamental vital fluids course in their normal state and quantity, accompanied by the normal processes of secretion, organic function, and intellection, is said to be a healthy person.

— SUSHRUTA-SAMHITA

Ayurveda teaches us that a healthy person is healthy in mind, body, and senses. We factor in what enters the body and how it is processed, utilized, and ultimately excreted. We evaluate actual food intake and anything else that comes in contact with the sense organs, such as sound, light, smells, and so on. Anything perceived by the senses is food.

We cannot deny that the mind and body are interconnected. When we feel physical pain, there are often mental symptoms that accompany this pain. When we feel stress, anxiety, anger, or sadness, we feel physical symptoms, too, because feelings trigger energy and fluids to travel differently through the body and can even cause muscle contractions or spasms.

A blood test can give us a view of how the various organs of the body are functioning in a moment of time. What a blood test cannot do is tell us how we feel, how hungry we are, or what thoughts we have. A blood test cannot teach us about the actual disease processes behind a snapshot in time. Ayurveda factors in all these things, because how we think, feel, and behave is certainly connected with how the body is operating. Health is really about ensuring that energy and fluids are flowing properly; the physical flow depends on mental and emotional flow, and vice versa. We must give importance to mental states, emotions, and the physical condition of the body equally.

Most people don't think too much about their health unless they've identified some sort of problem or discomfort in themselves. We also tend to think about our own health when a family member has a medical issue — we start to wonder if we will suffer the same fate due to genes, a similar diet, or a lifestyle that we have in common. Learning how to read the body on a day-to-day basis, and ultimately moment to moment, will actually help prevent health issues — even those we are predisposed to — because the cause of our imbalances can be determined sooner. This is why it's important to observe the condition of our physical attributes and physiological functioning on a regular basis, including:

- Body form and composition
- Skin, including scalp
- Tongue
- Eyes
- Nails

- Voice
- Urine
- Feces
- Bodily secretions (including reproductive-organ fluids and menstruation)

Physical forms change according to the volume, frequency, and type of energy they receive. Identifying issues with skin, digestion, or periods early is very important, because these can signal the first stages of imbalance and the start of a disease process. However, every woman has to get to know her body type at its best to understand what a balanced state feels like. For example, what is normal digestion? When I ask clients to tell me about their bowel movements, they oftentimes respond by saying they are normal or that they don't really look at them. This area of discussion is a bit embarrassing for a lot of people. In truth, "normal" is simply what a person is used to. It may or may not be a healthy state. Knowledge of Ayurveda helps a person identify the healthy state.

The Five Elements

To create anything, you need to know what materials you have at your fingertips.

Space, or *akasha*, is the first of the five elements Ayurveda uses to describe the matter we see in our bodies, in food, and in nature around us. Space provides a container for everything else, and even though we cannot see it — we know it's there because we can see what's in it. Our planet, the stars, and the sun are all in space. We can hear because sound travels through space. The body is essentially a collection of different types of channels (arteries, veins, organs, digestive tract, reproductive tract, bones, and so forth), and in each channel, there is a space for something to happen inside. Space exists in junction points, such as in the synapses between neurons and in joints. With too little space, congestion or inflammation happens, and with too much, things dry out or communications get dropped. Adequate space is a key to transmission — of information, nutrients, and energy. When a space suddenly opens up, a vacuum of receptivity is created. When a space is closed, transmission is blocked.

You can observe nature and see the same phenomena playing out in your own body. Sometimes just looking at a flower for a moment will tell you everything you need to know about how you feel right now. It may even help you solve a problem you've been working on. The space around us teaches us what is within us. This is because the atoms that make up the stars, the plants, and the ocean are the same atoms we have in our bodies. Creation, after all, is a reshuffling of matter and energy, and somewhere along the way, a new person like you or me comes into being.

Movement and change is created by **air**, or *vayu*. Like space, air is impossible to see, but we can see what it moves. We get our sense of touch from the air element, such as when we can feel the hairs on our arms move in the wind. A deficiency of air renders an organism inert, and excess can cause chaos and erosion. Air is necessary for respiration, for the wavelike movements of digestion (*peristalsis*), and for bodily and mental movements in general. We can have too much or too little air. Too little is lifeless; too much is degenerative.

Your Body's Wind Currents

After watching a meteorologist present weather patterns two or three times, you can see that some wind currents are common on our planet. Your body has some wind-current patterns as well. These are called the five vayus. Air travels in five general directions in a human body:

1. In and out with the breath — *prana vayu*
2. From the gut to the head to facilitate thinking and communication — *udana vayu*
3. In a linear fashion to balance pressure and deliver energy and nutrients across membranes — *samana vayu*
4. Downward with gravity and out through the digestive, reproductive, and urinary tracts — *apana vayu*
5. From the heart, through the blood vessels, to the entire periphery of the body — *vyana vayu*

All these vayus are important in order for you to feel fully alive. Certain vayus have a more dominant force at times, such as vyana vayu when your heart is pumping during cardiovascular exercise or a startled state, or apana vayu when you have your period. In fertility, apana vayu is an important wind current to study. A woman needs to allow some pull of gravity to feel stable, safe, and secure, but she must let apana vayu take over even more when menstruation begins. This is one of the reasons why women are not advised to practice handstands or other inversions in yoga class during menstruation. It's also a reason why women notice changes in their bowel movements around menstruation. The downward force is at play.

If a vayu becomes increased or blocked, it can affect other vayus by increasing or decreasing them. For example, a constipated person may find herself with health issues showing up in the upper part or periphery of the body, because if apana vayu has become blocked, then pressure will back up in the gut and this can push any toxicity into the blood, the lymph, and even the nerves. Also, if a person overexercises and increases energy taken in through the breath (prana), the preexisting imbalance patterns of each of the other vayus can increase even more.

Knowing that these wind currents exist, you can begin to direct energy mindfully throughout your body. You may have already noticed that some of these wind currents seem stronger than others. Your task is to seek out all the places in your body that may have become blocked so that you can let these currents flow freely—in just the right amounts for you to enjoy health and longevity.

Fire, or *tejas*, is responsible for transformation and provides heat, while our eyes perceive the light emitted from it. We need fire for body heat, proper digestion, and metabolism. Enzymes have fire in them to carry out their action. Too much fire element will burn (as in the case of hyperacidity or ulceration), and too little of it can cause slowness and stagnation. Extreme cases of low heat can also end up looking like burning tissues, as in frostbite, and an individual can have a burning sensation in the stomach when the body is too alkaline. The key is that the body needs a delicate balance of fire for metabolic purposes, and this balance is maintained by hunger, desire, bodily wastes, and excretions. The main fire tissues of the body are found in the liver, blood, and bile. Anemia signals an issue with an individual's fire element, as do the colors white, yellow, or red in the stool, skin, eyes, or tongue.

Hunger is desire, and desire is fire. Without desire, there would be no matter in the universe. Both desire and fire quicken movement. Heat makes water rise and evaporate. The result is lightness. When you're trying to create anything, fire gives objects their form, like a clay pot solidified in a hot oven. The positive transmutation of anger is passion and intensity. Do not hold in your fire. Find a way to lovingly escort it out toward a purpose that is greater than yourself so it does not damage your body.

The fourth element is **water**, or *jala*. Our planet is said to be made up of over 70 percent water, and our bodies have a lot of water, too. In the human body, water is responsible for lubrication, allowing mixing to occur, and maintaining temperature. Our tongues taste food because of water, and if we are dehydrated, our sense of taste can become affected. The many fluids of the body — plasma, lymph, cerebrospinal fluid, interstitial fluid, breast milk, and so on — all need water to be formed. Too little water prevents flow. Too much also prevents flow because it takes up too much space, causing pressure and diluting fire. All nutrients are transported in water.

When we are young, we are very juicy. Our bodies become drier the older we get. This causes the tissues to become less flexible and changeable. Very old people will often have large swatches of skin rip off because it has lost its moisture and has grown brittle, thin, and flaky. A baby is gestated in water. Water sustains life, but too much of it dulls the senses and fire element and dilutes potency. We can drink too little or too much, or imbibe at the wrong times.

The last and most tangible element is **earth**, or *prithvi*. Earth provides structure, coolness, and grounding. Our noses can smell the earth element, like the ground after a rain or the trees as we walk through the forest. We need earth for material form — our bodies need nourishment from the plants that grow on our planet. If we are meat eaters, the animals also get their nourishment from the plants. Too much earth will make us heavy and cold, and can create blockages and growths. Too little will waste away tissues and cause degeneration. All growth hormones include the earth element. We may feel a sense of lightness when we reduce the earth element, but too much lightening will then cause the body's functions to lose their integrity.

You are both an artist and a scientist. By noticing the five elements — space, air, fire, water, and earth — in all matter, you can direct and shift energies; your will becomes potent and effortless. When you have fire in the food you eat, you become fire. When you feel the air you breathe, you become air. When you stretch your arms out in a wide-open space, you become space. This is the poetry of the mind, body, and senses. This is Ayurveda.

Dosha Theory

Ayurvedic scholars of long ago discovered something really brilliant. They noticed that, despite the myriad physical and mental issues people have, all maladies can be grouped into only a handful of different categories of imbalance. The body displays these patterns through physiological signals, temperament, and behavior, but what's responsible for these displays is actually an imbalance of humors in the body. These humors are called *doshas* in Sanskrit. The word *dosha* literally means "that which can go out of balance."

These doshas produce both physiological and psychological symptoms. By their very nature, doshas are prone to going up and down in response to behavior, the environment, and the seasons. What we eat, sounds or smells we come in contact with, the weather, and even other people all affect our doshas because they each have unique properties that will either raise or lower a given dosha.

There are three doshas found in nature — *vata*, *pitta*, and *kapha* — and they are made up of the five elements previously covered. When a particular element increases, its corresponding dosha can increase. Similarly, when a particular element decreases, its linked dosha can decrease. If we haven't learned how to spot the signs of doshic imbalance, this is when problems occur. As we learn to balance our lives better, our doshas also become more balanced; and conversely, as we balance our doshas more, our lives become better.

Once you understand dosha theory, your life will be forever changed. You will see how doshas affect your body, mental state, emotions, and energy. You will observe and understand yourself with greater wisdom so you can prevent imbalances and heal quickly. Then you will become more present to the totality of life.

Vata (Space + Air)

The first dosha, *vata*, involves the elements of space and air and is difficult to see, but like the wind, it creates movement, dryness, roughness, chaos, and erosion. Individuals who have an excess of vata in their bodies would experience the qualities just described. They might feel extremely scattered, suffer from anxiety, and have difficulty sleeping. High-vata people are ungrounded, sometimes feeling wildly energetic. Too much vata causes rapid aging and degeneration. Vata naturally increases in older age, and it is increased prematurely with too much movement and travel. The wind blowing through you all the time can dry you out.

Vata is:

- Subtle
- Mobile
- Cold
- Dry

- Rough
- Light
- Clear
- Dispersing

Pitta (Fire + Water)

The second dosha, *pitta*, involves the fire and water elements. It's responsible for transformation, and it's what makes us a hot-blooded organism. Pitta can be found in the bile and in the blood, as well as in enzymes and processes that have a transforming nature. Pitta is like the lava of the body, and it increases with transformation. The result of too much pitta is inflammation. Red, rashy skin conditions, high acidity, jaundice, anger, sour smell, and yellow, loose stools are examples of too much pitta. A high-pitta person may feel hot, ambitious, managerial, and intense. She may want to wash her hair every day because it can get oily very quickly. She may like to wear makeup to cover up skin blemishes.

Pitta is:

- Hot
- Oily
- Light
- Sharp

- Fast
- Mobile
- Liquid

Kapha (Water + Earth)

The third dosha, *kapha*, is made of the water and earth elements. It provides the body with lubrication and structure, and you can recognize it in the form of mucus, saliva, and other bodily fluids, as well as in the meat and fat of the body. In excess, it can create heaviness and lethargy, manifesting as weight gain, frequent urination, nausea, and signs of prediabetes. Too much kapha shows up as cysts, tumors, and other types of growths. With high kapha, a person could feel stuck, stubborn, or overwhelmed by feelings of attachment.

Kapha is:

- Cool
- Wet
- Heavy
- Slow
- Slimy

- Dull
- Dense
- Static
- Cloudy

The following table explains the characteristics of each of the doshas and their relationship to the elements, plus what makes them increase and how to detect them.

CHARACTERISTICS OF THE THREE DOSHAS

DOSHA	ELEMENTS	FUNCTION	INCREASING FACTORS	ASSOCIATED SYMPTOMS
VATA	Space + air	Movement	Excessive intake of cold, dry, bitter, or astringent substances; travel; living off circadian rhythm; injury/worry	Degeneration: Dry tissues, twitching, anxiety, mania, poor memory, channel constriction, pain that travels around the body
PITTA	Fire + water	Transformation	Excessive intake of hot, oily, salty, sour, or pungent substances; hot, humid climates; working too much; anger	Inflammation: Red or oily tissues; allergies; baldness or early graying; heavy bleeding; red-blood-cell, liver, or spleen issues; fleshy smell
KAPHA	Water + earth	Nourishment	Excessive intake of cold, heavy, sweet, or salty substances; cool, cloudy, damp climates; laziness; attachment	Overnourishment: Swelling or increase of mucus or other fluids; tissue growths (tumors, cysts, skin tags); excessive hair growth; sweet, sticky blood; feeling of heaviness

Vata is actually known as the root of all other imbalances. When there is an excess of movement, any of the doshas can go out of balance fast. Vata can fuel the intensity of a person's fire, and it can also perpetuate overgrowth or aggravate clogging patterns.

Then, too, individuals can have more than one imbalanced dosha at the same time. When vata and pitta mix, the symptoms can really conflagrate because there is less moisture to protect. When pitta and kapha mix, the emotional states of anger and attachment can combine to create resentment and sourness.

In addition, despite the tendency for a woman to have a dominant dosha or two, different areas of her body can be experiencing an imbalance of different doshas. For example, externally a woman's skin can have rashes or red acne, a sign of excess pitta in the tissue, while her periods could appear scanty, or not at all, a sign of excess vata in the uterus. Or her digestion can show signs of dry constipation, an indicator of vata imbalance, while her periods may be very heavy, a sign of high pitta in the reproductive tissue. Because we are complex, it can take a while to sort ourselves out, especially if we are going it alone without the help of a practitioner, but starting with the basic understanding of the doshas is super helpful for most people.

Balancing the *Gunas*

Many women claim they want more balance, but they have difficulty articulating how to find this balance. Usually, they want to feel less stress. For a lot of modern women, less stress means less chaos or activity and more downtime or chill-out time. However, if a woman does not understand what is really causing her stress, then she will find that the same old stressors are there after she takes a break.

You have to get at the root cause of an imbalance for transformation to occur. It seems that many people understand this intellectually, but in order to truly get at the root cause, you have to gather the awareness around your mental, physical, and emotional dimensions of imbalance. Without all three, healing is incomplete.

When your body is hot, your mind can tend toward intensity, anger, or frustration. When you feel like you've been running around too much, the muscles can become tight because they've been trying to add resistance and gripping as you've been bouncing all over the place or trying to protect yourself. Then the tightness causes pain, which can make you *more* rigid and affect your physical and mental flexibility. When you finally get more rest — get grounded — your body relaxes. However, you still may not find balance, because you are simply getting a temporary reprieve from the perennial patterns creating the imbalances. This is where balancing with Ayurveda comes in.

Ayurveda looks at basic qualities in nature, referred to as *gunas*, when understanding the health of the body in an environment. You've probably heard the old saying "Opposites attract." A little different spin on that is found in one of the most important principles of Ayurvedic healing: *like increases like, and opposites balance each other.* To feel healthy, you need equilibrium in body, mind, senses, and emotions. Whenever you ingest a substance or come in contact with an object or person with properties similar to those residing within you, it increases those properties in you.

When a dosha gets out of balance, it is because there is disharmony in the balance of the gunas. However, we may only know that this problem exists when we see evidence of the dosha being imbalanced. This is why we study the doshas: to spot imbalance. Once we see that there is a doshic imbalance, we have to identify the gunas that are imbalanced.

Ten pairs of opposite qualities/gunas are looked at in evaluating health. These qualities may seem familiar because many of them are found in each of the doshas listed earlier.

Pairs of Opposite Qualities (Gunas)

- Hot — Cold
- Heavy — Light
- Oily — Dry
- Clear — Cloudy
- Slimy — Rough
- Gross — Subtle
- Mobile — Static
- Sharp/Fast — Dull/Slow
- Soft — Hard
- Dense — Liquid

Bodies naturally have certain characteristics, and sometimes we get too much of one of these qualities. For example, we may have skin that is on the oilier side, and occasionally it's off-the-charts oily. A woman in this situation has to wash her hair every day because she is so oily, whereas other women are so dry that they can go a whole week or even two without washing their hair. Some individuals are hot all the time, and others are cold all the time. Some women operate really quickly and tend to feel impatience, and others are a bit more laid-back and take their time — either because they move slowly or because they take a curvy line from point A to point B.

The gunas have physical and mental impacts. It's impossible to separate the mind from the body. Your existence encompasses both of these dimensions. When you have a psychological experience, it affects your body. When your body is affected, it affects your energy and ability to perceive the world accurately.

Opposite qualities can be used to balance overabundant qualities, so a person dealing with inflammation, a pitta issue from the hot guna, would benefit from being around cooling nature — plants, trees, and such — or drinking some sweet coconut water, but may get further out of balance by running a marathon in the summer heat. Learning how to play with opposites is the key to finding balance in life.

A woman may start to understand that life feels out of balance, and she can detect why and then rebalance with opposite qualities. For example, if she's out of balance because she's increased her mobility, getting way too busy, or because she's been spending too much time in a cold, dry environment, then she can counterbalance with slowness and grounding, warming, and hydrating herself. If she's been working super frantically and in fast mode for extended periods of time, then she can counterbalance with slowness and dullness. If she's been eating too many cloudy foods, like dairy or nut-milk products, making her system feel foggy or clogged, then she can start to balance that with foods that are clear instead.

Balancing the opposites artfully and in the right amounts is key. We don't want the pendulum to swing in another direction, because we can then create another imbalance of the opposite quality. For instance, if we try to balance cloudiness with clarity and go overboard, then there will be no resistance, and life still needs a little resistance.

EXERCISE: IDENTIFYING YOUR IMBALANCED GUNAS

Bring your awareness to your life, body, or a specific part of it that feels imbalanced for you, and note which of the twenty gunas/qualities feel significantly noticeable. Note these qualities down somewhere.

Next, call to mind the opposite quality that could balance out each of the excess qualities that you have noted. Note these opposite qualities next to the excess qualities.

Artfully balancing the opposites is one way you can tap back into your body's primal, animal power — and improve your health in the process — simply by honoring nature. Your health does not have to be so complicated!

(Keep your pen and paper or journal handy, as I will ask you to take some more notes later on.)

Honoring Circadian Rhythms

Humans are not sleeping the way nature intended.
The number of sleep bouts, the duration of sleep, and when sleep
occurs have all been comprehensively distorted by modernity.

— MATTHEW WALKER,
Why We Sleep: Unlocking the Power of Sleep and Dreams

When I started practicing Ayurveda, I noticed that the people with the worst constipation and irritable-bowel-type digestion also had the most abnormal sleeping behaviors, and some would not believe me when I told them that there is a correlation between living off from the circadian rhythms and having poor digestion and health. For most of my own life, I've been a superb sleeper, but I experienced firsthand after having a child how sleep deprivation affects physiology. It may be difficult to make the connection, but *when* you sleep, wake, and nap all have a huge effect on you. Daily and seasonal cycles have an impact on both mind and body.

Ayurvedic medicine has been teaching for centuries how sleeping and eating in line with nature's rhythms is necessary for optimal health, and modern medicine is also now advocating more strongly for this idea. In 2017, the Nobel Prize in Physiology or Medicine was actually awarded to a team of researchers who found scientific evidence of the molecular mechanisms that attune organisms' bodies to day/night cycles for optimal functioning. Good sleep and timing activities according to the sun and moon cycles are absolute necessities for good health. All lifestyle misdeeds affect the body, and any lack of health in the body can affect the reproductive functioning. Interestingly, the specific amount of sleep a woman needs depends on her constitution, life stage, and lifestyle.

Biologically, humans, like most other species, are patterned to be somewhat ritualistic in their behavior. The natural calls of the sun and the moon and the stars are there for all of us, but as inventions and advancements in technology allow us to keep our world lit up at night, many people find themselves either working at odd times or simply staying up to read, watch videos, or party way after the sun has gone down. Some carry into adulthood an almost childlike desire to rebel against their parents' bedtime rules, which they start to self-impose as adults. They do not want to hear that they have to go to bed at a decent time, because to them it feels like an arbitrary rule, but it is important to do if they actually want to be healthy. They may say they can't sleep unless they take something, but taking a medicine to fall asleep is only a short-term solution that makes the problem worse if it becomes part of the regular routine. The issue will persist as long as the cause preventing a person from being able to sleep is not identified and removed. The same principle applies for any imbalance of body and mind.

The Ayurvedic Clock

Ayurveda has taught that the time when an individual goes to bed, eats meals, and tries to perform different sorts of activities matters greatly. The Ayurvedic clock breaks the day into six circadian segments that follow nature's cycles. Each segment has dominant energies, which will either support an activity or make it more challenging.

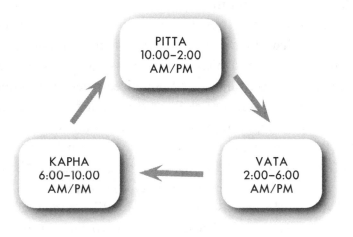

Figure 3: The Ayurvedic clock

KAPHA TIME OF DAY

This time of day — 6:00–10:00 AM and 6:00–10:00 PM — is the naturally grounded, cooling, calm part of the day, when life either has not gotten busy yet or has started to settle down back to the earth. The slow heaviness of the night's sleep has not completely worn off in the morning's kapha phase, and the activity and chaos of the day is decreasing in the evening's kapha phase. These two times of day are good to indulge in more sleep if an individual is burned-out or depleted, but if issues have arisen from overnourishment or heaviness, then it's best to be moving during this time of the day.

Individuals who eat during the kapha times of day will build tissues more than people who do so during other times of day. Those who sleep too much at this time will find they have difficulty getting moving — they will feel lethargy and heaviness. Those who are burned-out or dried-out may feel they have more stamina during kapha time.

Pitta Time of Day

This interval — 10:00–2:00 AM and 10:00–2:00 PM — is the more heating, energized time of day. People have typically gotten into their workday and have found that they are productive and active. It's the time when the digestive strength is generally strongest, which is good for those who have lunch in the middle of their day, but for people who stay up after ten at night, this can also be tricky because they will often start to get hungry and energized when they should have already gotten themselves to sleep before the fire energy rises again. This is especially important when there is a full moon and individuals get struck with the extra energy of all the added light rays bouncing around. More light stimulates the pitta of the eyes, and the eyes are directly connected to the rest of the nervous system.

Individuals who exercise during the pitta time of day will find they have lots of energy for it. Those who are burned-out, though, would be best served by avoiding exercise during this time of day and be better off doing some gentle yoga or tai chi or even taking a brief post-lunch nap instead of being active.

Vata Time of Day

This time of day — 2:00–6:00 AM and 2:00–6:00 PM — is the period of movement and space. In the morning, since most creatures are sleeping during this time, there is much empty space, but soon nature begins to stir and the day's movement begins. During this time in the morning, the birds start to chirp, and many individuals find themselves waking from their sleep, if only briefly. The afternoon vata period, too, is thought of as the time when the workday's intensity starts to quiet down, and the spaciousness can open up creativity. But soon afterward the afternoon commute begins for many people as they transition to evening routines.

Finding Your Own Normal within Your Environment

When we don't pay attention to how our bodies are functioning on a day-to-day basis, diseases seem to come out of nowhere, and we cannot understand how they were created. It sometimes seems difficult to connect certain behaviors to how the body is functioning, or not functioning. We don't always notice the effects because we may be mentally scattered; too tired; or simply focused on something else altogether, like work, family, or relationships — even the news can occupy our minds so much that we don't pay attention to our bodies.

I recall in my earliest days of doing Ayurvedic consultations that many people expressed to me that they did not look in the toilet after they went to the bathroom unless they had some sort of serious digestive issue. I would ask them to describe what their bowel movements looked like — color, shape, texture, size, number of pieces — and many would not have an answer, as I mentioned previously, or they would simply say something like "I don't know…normal." The problem is that *normal* does not exist, and the details matter when it comes to observing the body.

Talking about bowel movements can sometimes be uncomfortable for people because we've been conditioned to be embarrassed by this normal, natural bodily function. However, Ayurveda requires gaining life knowledge, so if you look at even the things that are embarrassing, then you have more information about your life that could really help you heal imbalances. Looking at what's in the toilet was one of the first things we were taught in Ayurveda school. It actually becomes fascinating and even fun once you get into it.

All the body's excretions tell us how it processed what went in. We can learn about moisture, metabolic strength and speed, and whether we are making the right choices for our body type and season. This information is invaluable, because it teaches us that small differences on a day-to-day basis affect our health.

Like bodily excretions, sleep is also a basic life function that often does not get enough attention, but it has a huge impact on people's mental and physiological functioning. Many people wake up in the morning not feeling rested. Some know it's because they did not get enough sleep, but others are unaware that they may have actually gotten *too much*, and that is causing lethargy. Yes, a person can actually get too much sleep and still feel tired. In those cases, the solution is not to sleep more but to get the body moving — walking briskly, running, or doing some other exercise. There is an ideal amount of sleep for each of us.

Choose to go through your life not just existing but *thriving*. When you make good choices, your actions will result in favorable outcomes and you will have vitality. You can see how the environment affects you and how you affect the environment. To thrive, you need to give your body the foods, sleep, and other sensory inputs that help you feel your best.

You have to prioritize the functioning of your body, mind, and spirit very highly — even if you feel this is difficult because other people are relying on you. Perhaps it's work, family, friends, your partner — or, later, your children — distracting you from being able to take care of yourself. However, developing the art of self-care is important in order for you to be of good service to anyone in the long term. If *you* do not focus on this, no one will do it for you.

There is no perfect ideal to strive toward. Rather, there is simply a nonstop balancing act (that is, homeostasis) that the body is usually aware of but which sometimes the mind overrides because it's gotten conditioned into thinking that life is supposed to be a certain way that is not actually biologically or mentally helpful to us. This conditioning comes from our parents, teachers, jobs, peers, and lovers; the government; advertising; and even our own egos. By studying how the body is being affected, we are very quickly brought back to reality, and then we can surrender to the fact that sometimes our minds are making poor choices, even when we think we are being so smart.

Align your intellect, body, and desire, and you will thrive. Do not allow yourself to get stuck in thoughts that aren't real, even if they seem real. Do not hold in your fear, anger, resentment, clinging, greed. Do not get set in your ways at the expense of your body. Be bold. Study your body to see if your decisions are working out for you. You have choices about how to live your life, and the time for you to exercise them is now — especially if you are thinking about becoming a mother.

In the next chapters, I'll discuss how to care for your body, how to read what's being brought in through the senses, and how to create a state of passionate receptivity and resiliency, which is necessary for any sort of creation.

Chapter 4

The Four Fertility Factors

The upwelling of the sea continues.

— BRENDA HILLMAN, "A Spiral Tries to Feel Again"

A woman with an optimally functioning body has the ability to conceive and birth a child with a suitable partner during the fertile years of her life. If there is no intervention, it's possible for her to get pregnant from a very young age all the way until she finally goes through menopause. Fertility increases when the conditions in the environment are conducive to the creation and growth of a child, and these conditions can differ case by case because each baby has its unique nature, or *prakruti*, as does each mother and father. This is the biological norm. No two are the same. Modern medicine refers to the genome, which is a part of prakruti.

Today, modern women are very concerned about the environment, whether this be the stress level in the place where they work, the state of political affairs, or even literally the condition the earth is in. We see people headed out to explore the possibility of bringing life out into space, and we start to wonder whether it could really be so bad down here on Earth that we feel the need to leave the planet.

Ayurveda creates a natural harmony by connecting a person's inner world (the mind, body, and spirit) with the outer world (the seasons, environment, and larger macrocosm). Ayurveda does this by preventing and reversing disease, improving quality of life, and increasing longevity for the individual's unique constitution, and it has been doing so for thousands of years. It is absolutely possible to tip the balance toward health, even in a shifting environment.

Furthermore, the ancient wisdom of Ayurveda brings us back to the very simple biological ideas behind how life is created. There are Four Fertility Factors to consider for natural fertility and reproductive health: *seed*, *season*, *field*, and *water*.

1. **Seeds** are the ovum and sperm that join together and get implanted in the uterus. Seeds are also the intentions a woman has for supporting another life on the planet. They are given a chance only when the conditions are right for them to grow in.

2. **Season** is synonymous with timing: time of life, time of year, monthly cycle, and day. There are optimal times for each woman to have a child.

3. **Field** includes the uterus and other reproductive organs, which contribute to the creation and gestation of a fetus and the nurturing of a child, as well as the larger environment around mother, child, and family. The field is a welcoming home for a new baby.

4. **Water** is what flows through the field to nourish tissues of both mother and child, delivering messages via hormones and lubricating the body for the immense physical changes taking place during the menstrual cycle, gestation, and birth. The water element is a nurturer, a carrier, and a mixer. It maintains the stability of the temperature inside the body so that metabolic processes can take place within their optimum range.

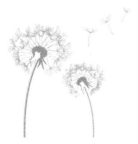

Seed = Oocyte, sperm. These join together and are planted inside the woman's uterus to grow.

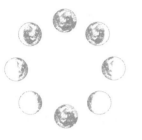

Season = Time of life, month, or year. The menstrual cycle, biological clock, and cyclical rhythms of nature all sync up for divine conception to occur.

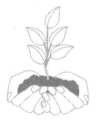

Field = The woman's body, partner, and environment. The uterus, follicles, ovary, and fallopian tubes; one's parents and lover; and the community are all working together to bring forth new life.

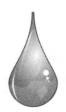

Water = Hormones, amniotic fluid, vaginal fluid, and pregnancy swelling. Liquid nourishes and lubricates the great changes that take place in creation.

Figure 4: The Four Fertility Factors

If there is trouble in any of these four fertility areas, conception may become challenging. Mind, body, and environment are all important considerations on the path to getting pregnant. Your partner and larger community environment factor in, but you are prime. You make decisions about whom to bring into your life, what to put into your body, when to explore having a family, and which career choices to make.

To influence the fertility factors, Ayurveda focuses on optimizing a person's day-to-day routines, diet, and lifestyle with self-care and attunement to the environment. You plant your seeds, and at the right time, in the right environment, and with the right care — you might start "sprouting" a baby. However, the goal here is not just to get pregnant. You also want the rest of your life and health to be going well. Your health is one of the greatest gifts you can give to anyone, including yourself, your partner, and potentially your future baby.

If you have physical issues with your cycles or other key areas of the body, or any mental turbulence about having a child, then it's time to make healing decisions. It is important to work on resolving chronic issues before you conceive. You want to be in the best health possible when you embark on the path to motherhood because, while it's possibly the most rewarding experience in a woman's life, it's not a walk in the park. Pregnancy and motherhood can make certain physical and mental health conditions worse for some women and even pass on the condition to their unborn babies. For example, a woman with cancer is at risk of the cancer worsening during pregnancy, and it's also possible for some cancers to spread to the fetus in utero.

Luckily, when babies are born today, generally things seem to develop quite well. Most babies are born with all their parts intact, as only 3 percent suffer any type of major birth defect whatsoever. It turns out that nature is successful in building bodies without much conscious help from us!

Much like a garden, one's fertility can be cultivated in a natural way with some time and attention. Through identifying the Four Fertility Factors, you will be able to create a healthy, rewarding, and beautiful experience for yourself and your family.

Let's go into these fertility factors a little more deeply so you can nurture your health and develop more trust in the wisdom of the body.

Seed

If you look at a strawberry, you can see a whole bunch of seeds on it. A strawberry is actually the ovary of the strawberry plant. Its sole purpose is reproduction, though we humans love it because it tastes so sweet and so tart and makes us salivate. It stains our teeth and tongue red for a moment before all its deliciousness goes down into the digestive tract. Our ovaries are a bit like strawberries — they have a rounded shape as well, and their purpose is to house all the seeds we have to bring to the reproductive table until it's time for them to be released into the wild.

The Great Incubator

Most women have two ovaries — one attached to either side of the uterus (the central organ of the reproductive system) via a ligament, a type of connective tissue. The ovary is essentially an olive-shaped incubator of a woman's eggs. From the environment, it receives cues to promote or inhibit growth, as well as nourishment to build the quality of its cells. The outer layer of the ovary is called the *germinal epithelium*, and it's essentially like a type of skin. Under that layer is a layer of connective tissue, and then the inner body of the ovary contains both a *cortex* (a supportive outer tissue housing the cells that become your eggs) and a *medulla* (inner connective tissue containing nerves and blood vessels). If these terms sound a little familiar, it's because your brain and several other organs have both a cortex and a medulla as well. It turns out that nature likes to repurpose formats where it can, even though it does other strange things that are difficult to understand at times! Could it be that your ovaries are as smart as your brain?

Creating Eggs Before We Are Born

One such strange thing the female body does is prepare way in advance for having children. In fact, modern science says that all the potential eggs a woman will ever have in her ovaries are deposited in that organ while she is still in her mother's belly! Most men, on the other hand, do not start producing their seed until they reach puberty. In both cases, the seeds are created by each person's body; it's just that the woman's seeds are produced while someone else is making conscious decisions about what gets inside her body: her mother. A woman pregnant with a daughter is, at the same time, cocreating her potential daughter's eggs to be used in the future. The final product of this work in the female fetus is called the *primary oocyte*, and it gets deposited into the ovary for safekeeping as a primordial follicle (an immature oocyte with some epithelial cells around it) until the fertile years and a particular menstrual cycle calls it into action. An oocyte can be created as many as fifty-some years before it actually becomes fully mature and is given a chance at conception!

Just think about this for a moment. Cells are formed based on the nutrients received, metabolic capacity, and the balances of energies present at the time of their creation. So a mother has a fair amount of influence over the health of her daughter's potential babies, since the seeds are planted while she is still in the womb, when Mama is feeding her via the umbilical cord. If you are happy with your health, then perhaps you'd better take the time to thank not only your mama for growing you inside her belly but also *her* mama for having a hand in your original creation. And if you have seeds in your ovaries, then both you and your mother are to thank for building those.

At the same time that we should be thanking our mamas and grandmas, we should also be recognizing how much our entire lives affect our eggs. We are a little different from men in this regard, because a man's sperm are thought to regenerate indefinitely, while a woman's oocytes are believed to be unable to regenerate. This effectively means that what a woman gets before she is born is all she will have available to her, which is one reason why so many women feel the pressure of the biological clock so intensely, while men don't seem as concerned: women are essentially born with a reproductive bank account opened by their mothers that collects no interest, and some of what was initially deposited gets spent every month — but men open their own bank account when they hit puberty and can keep getting returns on the initial investments they put into it.

Risks with Advanced Maternal Age

While it may seem unfair that men can have kids longer, nature actually has a smart reason to shorten the fertility window for women. The body is less able to withstand change and physical trauma as it gets older — and growing and bearing a child is the ultimate change for a woman's body. Many women of a more advanced age who are considering motherhood develop concern about their child potentially having birth defects, but they must also take into account their own health and resilience!

Women who give birth at an older age are at a higher risk for preeclampsia, gestational diabetes, *placenta previa* (part of the placenta growing over the cervix), *vasa previa* (baby's abnormal blood vessels blocking the cervix), and non–medically necessary C-sections (and C-sections cause a whole other set of health issues). Their children are at greater risk for having low birth weight, preterm births, and lower Apgar scores, which measure a baby's basic physical and physiological health at birth.

Don't Play the Numbers Game

When women begin to look into their fertility, many of them want to know how many eggs they have left. This is, unfortunately, not a number that a woman can actually obtain while she is alive and her ovaries are inside her, but she can get proxies for this information. There are blood tests available to test follicle-stimulating hormone (FSH), which is the hormone coming from the anterior part of the pituitary gland (in the brain) to the follicles to trigger growth. Blood tests for anti-Mullerian hormone (AMH), secreted by cells in the follicle, tell a woman the degree of follicle growth occurring as a response to the FSH. And there is a blood test for luteinizing hormone (LH), which also comes from the anterior pituitary, like FSH, but signals the ovaries to release an egg from the ovary.

However, importantly, none of these blood tests will tell a woman how many eggs she has left or whether she can get pregnant. Rather, when hormonal testing is conducted, a doctor may *infer* the number of eggs. Nonetheless, women seem to want this data when they decide they want to have a child. They want to know how they stack up — what their odds are. For many women, hard data can give peace of mind — for others, it will drive them nuts.

While it is generally known that follicle growth decreases with age, women today place too much focus on the numbers. Women don't need so many follicles to develop to maturity. They need only one to be released during ovulation. Therefore, as long as a woman is ovulating, then the possibility for pregnancy is still there. It is not healthy to become obsessed with how many eggs are left, how many follicles are growing, and the like, because this can cause great distress and possibly make the fertility journey a miserable one. Once a woman begins to stress out, believing she is not as fertile as she once was, this can lead to rash decisions.

For natural conception, it's more important to focus on the factors influencing your fertility than it is to try to change your fertility directly. This requires a deep focus on your own health — physical, mental, and emotional. If you cultivate health the Ayurvedic way, then you will get pregnant if the conditions are right for it.

Case Study: Wanting a Baby, Looking for a Partner

My client Amber was thirty-nine and wanted to have a child in the future. When she came to me for fertility preparation, she was exploring all options available to her. She was concerned about her egg quality at her age, and especially about whether she'd be able to have a biological child.

She was dating, but none of the relationships were serious enough for her to want to have a baby with any of the men. She was clear that she didn't want to have a child without a stable partner yet didn't seem to be ready to settle down with someone because she was dating guys in other relationships or guys who lived very far from where she did. She had been wanting to find a good partner for a long time, but she was having little luck, despite being an attractive, educated woman. She was a busy person and very focused on her career. She was inflexible with her schedule and had difficulty forming deep, meaningful relationships because her interactions were often brief and action-oriented. She had trouble getting vulnerable with people, and being so obsessed with her work and personal interests, she allowed no space for a relationship.

When she came to me for help, she wanted to do an Ayurvedic cleanse. She had been on the pill for many years and wanted to be sure all the added hormones were completely out of her. At the same time, she was contemplating whether it was worth it to freeze her eggs in case she didn't find a partner for a few more years, assuming that her egg quality would be better now, at her current age, than when she actually found a partner. This got her interested in the idea of knowing her egg count.

I have encountered similar situations a lot. I explained to Amber that even after running tests, she wouldn't know her actual egg count or get any guarantees that she'd be able to have a biological child, but she could get some directional information. Even science has limitations when it comes to making things happen. However, when the mind is active, sometimes the only way to stop its speculations is to get some hard data — even if it's not answering one's specific question.

Luckily, Amber had a body type that visibly and functionally didn't seem to be aging very rapidly. Her tissues were of a robust and juicy quality. On the other hand, she had signs of blockage and overnourishment in her body. We worked together to put her on a lightening therapy (or *langhana*) that consisted of fasting and cleansing herbs and yoga practices.

She decided not to freeze her eggs, and after making several key lifestyle shifts, including working less, nourishing less frequently, and getting more in touch with her deep-seated emotions so they could be released, she met a new partner. In that healing space, she was able to release toxins she had been holding on to for a long time. With Ayurvedic treatment, her body became more receptive, and emotionally, she was able to more intimately connect with her new partner. The two of them conceived a child naturally when she was forty-one years old.

There is no correct answer when it comes to whether you should do testing. At thirty-eight I personally ran my FSH and LH just to satisfy my own curiosity because I was so concerned about my age and my partner not being ready to have a child yet. You will need to do what satisfies your mind, your heart, and your reproductive system — do what you need to do to get them in sync. However, do not let biomarkers lock you into a reality. If you find the hormonal balances are off and you want to get pregnant naturally, take steps to realign your health and environment first rather than running straight to fertility treatments.

Because the brain is involved in sending hormones to the reproductive organs, your conscious thoughts must be mined. For example, the purpose of FSH is to stimulate follicles that have eggs in them, and the purpose of LH is to release the egg from the follicle and ovary. Neither of these hormones tells the egg to create a baby. They simply are trying to make the egg available and healthy. Nature has to do the rest. Therefore, when a woman thinks too much about her goal of becoming pregnant, which is one possible end result of a menstrual cycle, there are a bunch of steps in between that are possibly not getting the attention they need — such as making the egg available, waiting for Mr. Right's sperm to reach it, letting the sperm in, giving time for the egg and sperm to create a zygote, carrying the zygote to the uterus, and then allowing it to implant there. It is best to be patient and allow these steps to happen if you want to get pregnant naturally.

If you were an animal in the wild, you would just get it on and not worry about the consequences, but you have a really smart mind — and you have access to medical testing, which animals do not. Many women do not have any fertility testing done. They simply go on how their bodies feel. However, if you have fear or doubt, sometimes tests can be helpful to ease your mind. When your mind is at ease, you can pay more attention to your body.

As long as the mind is thinking, peace is hard to find! And as long as you are grasping or forcing, you don't have peace of mind. Do what you need to do to let your mind rest. There is no fixed path. But whatever you choose, remember that numbers represent a snapshot in time and can actually be changeable.

While it is more ideal in many cases to have a child when you are younger, this is not what happens for many women. Many women over thirty-five, forty, and sometimes even forty-five have children (though the latter is very rare). At the time I was pregnant, I grew close with several other women who were having babies. Two of these women were thirty-six, two were forty-three, and one was a few days shy of forty-eight when each had her first child. We all had generally healthy pregnancies and babies. I am not advocating for waiting to have children. In fact, I advocate for having them much younger than I did, but you should know that it's possible for many women to have healthy children even later in their fertile years, though it comes with more likelihood of complications with both getting pregnant and delivering.

While it can feel overwhelming for a woman to find out her follicle-emitted AMH levels are low, sometimes crushing any expectation she had of having children, it is important to know that nature also does weird things sometimes and surprises us. One woman's AMH numbers were so low that her fertility doctor wouldn't agree to attempt any IVF treatments on her. She gave up on the prospect of ever having a child, and then right before she turned forty, she found out that she had a pretty crazy cyst that was interfering with ovulation. She had the cyst removed, ovulation picked back up again, and she had a surprise pregnancy years after completely abandoning hope. Moral of the story: take care of you first, and miracles can happen.

It is also important to note that women are all aging at different rates, depending on their birth constitution, lifestyle, and environment. One woman's thirty-six is another woman's thirty-one. If you don't see signs of aging in other tissues of your body, especially in your skin, then you might possibly be one of the women who don't age as quickly. The next section, "Season," will outline some of the signs of aging so you can get a feel for how likely you are to have degenerating fertility. Don't just assume you are like everyone else. Develop confidence by studying your own body Ayurvedically, so you don't have to cling to test results or pray for a miracle.

Season

A woman's fertility is governed by timing. Whether it's determining when in life to have a child or getting the phase right in the menstrual cycle to either promote or prevent pregnancy, time is a major factor. Even the time of year can have an impact on fertility, because the climate and environment affect the condition of our bodies. We share so many similarities with the plants and flowers — we each have our best seasons to grow in. Every woman should understand the basic patterns that women go through, but we must also learn about our unique constitution, because certain aspects of our health can fall outside of norms, medians, and averages and still be perfectly normal and healthy.

Life Stages

Everything created starts as something subtle and then turns into something gross, and once it becomes gross, it again turns into something subtler. Such is the arc of human life. We begin from a seed, perhaps even as an idea or a feeling before that, and then we turn into a full-fledged human body, only to break down again to give all our elements back to the earth.

Bodies are more watery and earthy when they are younger. In middle age, the body becomes more fiery, and then in older age, things become a little less material as the air and space elements take over. Because transformation requires fire, the middle part of life is when a woman reproduces, while she is in her active, fertile years. Her transformative powers are greatest in this phase of life.

More water means more lubrication, and lubrication helps you withstand great change. If you are going to push something the size of a butternut squash through an apple-size hole (the cervix should dilate to ten centimeters in diameter before a woman begins pushing), then you really, really want to make sure your tissues are juicy, lubricated, and able to tolerate that sort of pressure and trauma. In the later fertile years, the water element begins to decrease, and this causes a decrease in the lubricating properties of the body, as well as hormonal interruption.

Once a woman hits menopause, and the air and space elements begin to reduce the material nature of the body, reproductive functioning ends — thankfully so, because can you imagine gaining twenty to fifty pounds, and the damage caused by pushing a baby out once your tissues have become less robust and pliable?

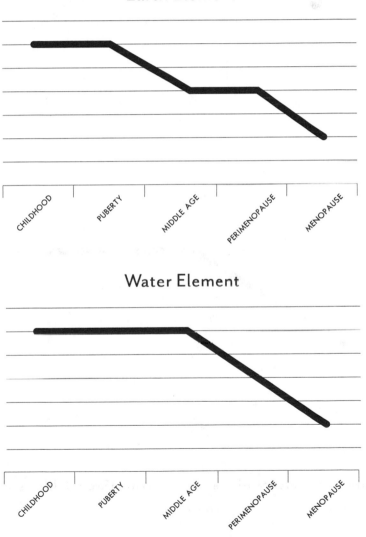

Figure 5: Prevalence of the five elements through life's stages

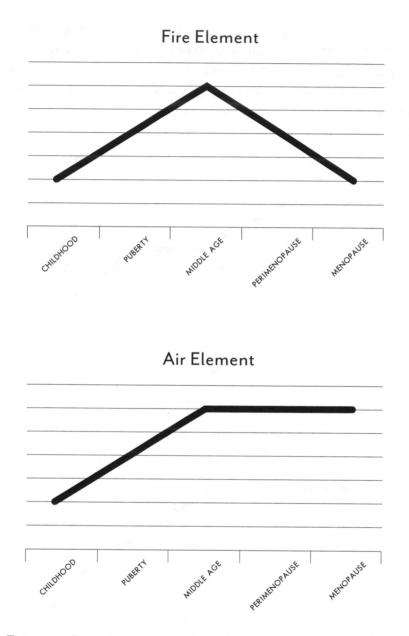

Figure 5: Prevalence of the five elements through life's stages
(continued)

Space Element

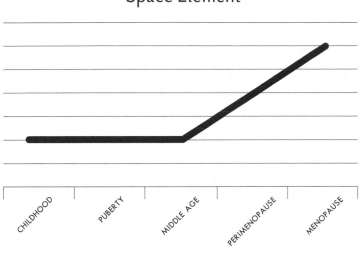

Figure 5: Prevalence of the five elements through life's stages
(continued)

As you can see, there is not one perfect time for a woman to have a child — it really depends on her unique situation. Fortunately, most women's water and earth elements do not take a sharp decline until menopause. Women with a vata imbalance may find their water element declining early, and those with a kapha imbalance may find theirs declining later. Women dealing with inflammatory pitta issues while trying to conceive or carry the child may find these issues exacerbated during pregnancy because the fire element increases dramatically during gestation. Understanding the common tendencies women face during certain life stages is very helpful, but understanding your unique constitution is even more important.

Seasonal Patterns

Bodily tissue quality, physiological functioning, and mood are all affected by the seasons of the year. Temperature, humidity, air pressure, wind, sunlight, and hours of daylight change constantly, but patterns are found in each of the seasons. A person's body constitution may operate more effectively in certain seasons and times of the year. One need only look to the gunas of a particular season. Bodies are wetter in warm, rainy seasons. People typically get "colds" more when the days are shorter, with less sunlight, and the temperature drops. Winter can be cold and dry in many areas, and any exposed tissues on the body can become rough. Hot weather tends to increase rashes.

All tissues of the body can be subject to the effects of the seasons. If you look at your life from year to year, you may notice that there are certain seasons when you feel healthier and others when you seem to get out of balance more. Learning about your Ayurvedic constitution can be beneficial, because it will give you tools for balancing your body seasonally.

Seasonal changes are not something happening to you only. They affect everyone. Ayurveda teaches that late winter/early spring, being kapha season, is typically the time when bodies are most robust. Late spring/summer is considered pitta season, when nature is the most intense and transformative. Fall/early winter, vata season, is when nature develops a sense of lightness, clarity, and spaciousness. There are slight nuances, depending on the unique climate in which you live. Later in this book, you may find considering the seasonal tendencies to be helpful in observing the patterns that your body and menstrual cycles exhibit.

Seasonal Transitions

Since each season has its own qualities, changing our diet and lifestyle seasonally is a must-do regular practice. If we do not eat what grows seasonally and notice the qualities that are changing in nature around us, then we can cause our bodies and minds to go out of balance. Our bodies get accustomed to the food and weather we experienced during the previous season. New qualities will begin to accumulate in nature and in the body in the next season. Adapting our diet and lifestyle helps prevent doshas from accumulating, aggravating, and causing disease. In addition, because a woman will conceive in one season and give birth in a completely different season, she has to be able to read her environment to make sure both she and her baby are healthy.

Seasonal transitions, referred to as *ritusandhi*, or the point at which one season meets the next, are periods of balancing opportunity. Oftentimes they are intervals when a person will notice that the dominant dosha from the previous season has gone out of balance. Some changes are typically necessary during these periods for health to be maintained. Best practices for your body at this time include changing diet and lifestyle to those appropriate for the coming season — slowly, within a couple of weeks. If a dosha got out of balance in the previous season, then it may naturally balance out in the upcoming one, or it may get worse.

This is where the idea of seasonal cleanses and seasonal eating comes from. The seasonal transitions are the period when, similar to knowing the market events that are good for buying and selling stocks, you either develop new health routines or drop old ones. If you continue to fail to see the qualities changing in nature around you, following old routines, then problems may occur. Waiting too long to change your routines will cause more problems. Ritusandhi is the opportunity to adjust behavior *before* problems due to environment/climate changes get out of hand and become too difficult to balance.

DOSHAS BY SEASON

SEASONAL JUNCTION	DOSHA TYPICALLY BUILDING IN THIS SEASON	DOSHA THAT MAY HAVE ACCUMULATED IN THE PREVIOUS SEASON
Late winter / early spring	Kapha	Vata
Late spring / summer	Pitta	Kapha
Fall / early winter	Vata	Pitta

Holidays and yearly work cycles for certain careers can also affect the mental and physical health of a woman. Say you have a very busy time during budgeting season in the fall because you work in finance, or you have to travel a lot in January because it's when your sales season kicks up. While these are not nature's rhythms, they are part of your seasonal lifestyles that you must consider when balancing your health.

Healthy Tissues and Signs of Aging

Why is it that some women seem to age faster than others? Some remain able to have children longer, while others find their ovarian reserve is depleted much earlier than they would have expected. Aging is a normal biological process, but it happens at different rates for different people. Part of this is the constitution we are born with, and the other part is how we manage our lifestyle.

As we covered earlier in this book, a human body's life has a building phase, a maintenance phase, and a breakdown phase. Aging occurs when a tissue begins to break down past its maintenance levels. Wrinkles, gray hair, thinning skin, memory issues, and muscle loss are examples of aging. While time is a factor in aging, lifestyle matters very much, too. Anytime a tissue gets depleted and does not get rejuvenated adequately afterward, the body is at risk of aging. Tissues get depleted when nutrition is improper or if there is poor digestion and assimilation due to metabolic issues. Partially this is because the body is not getting what its specific life demands call for, and partially it is because what is actually being ingested is starting to form toxins in the body and block nutrients from getting to the places they are needed.

To maintain healthy tissues, following an Ayurvedic diet and lifestyle protocol is necessary. This means throwing out the fad diets — all the things you heard were healthy for people — and really looking at what your specific body requires in order to meet the needs of your lifestyle. Issues with metabolism, growths of any sort, hormonal imbalances, inflammation, immune disorders, and depletion are calls for attention. A body aging quickly likely is in need of very delicate cleansing and rejuvenation. A healthy woman is one who has healthy tissues. She has balanced energy, a radiant glow, and a strong immunity. If a woman doesn't have these markers of health, she needs therapies to restore her vitality and immunity, referred to in Ayurveda as *rasayana* therapies.

Getting real about the state of your health is important, period. But it's even more important to have optimal health if you are considering getting pregnant. If you were a baby, wouldn't you prefer to enter into a healthy, resilient environment, rather than a toxic one? There is no better way to create a good environment in your body than to get on board with the present moment. That's the best clock to align with.

Field

When the body is ready to become pregnant, it sends signals. Depending on how much you pay attention to your body, you may or may not notice them. Taking care of your body and having a child are both a bit like taking care of a plant, except your *body* is where the seeds are planted, rather than the soil. Many women claim that they can't keep a plant alive. I've been one of these women. It's actually not that hard to keep a plant alive with a little bit of time and attention, but if we busy ourselves with other things, we will miss seeing what a plant needs to live.

I always purchased plants that were low-maintenance so that I could live my busy lifestyle without having to worry much about them. I did well with cacti, of course, and fine with a ficus — basically anything that didn't require a ton of watering or attention. Air plants were a dream, because I could completely neglect them and they'd be fine. Once I found a suitable spot in my apartment, I would water my plants once or twice a week. They did not grow much. They grew, but they didn't grow well. I assumed this was because I had bought them at IKEA or something like that, so they weren't very good plants. I never connected their growth to my behavior.

One day I decided I wanted to try my hand at outdoor plants, so I went to the garden store and stocked my deck full of mostly succulents, which I was told were typically the best for the environment and how infrequently I assumed I'd water them with my busy work schedule. I also selected one plant that was a little bit of a risk because I loved how it looked so much, a "red apple" aptenia. I had seen this plant thrive as ground cover and was told it might not do well where I was going to plant it, hanging from a planter on my deck. But I fell in love with this plant, and ignoring the wisdom shared with me, I bought a ton of it and draped it from my balcony, unsupported, in the hot sun.

The first two weeks were fine, but after that, I could see that this environment was clearly not working for the plant, even when I tried to water it more. It didn't seem to die, but it was just chugging along and looked like it was undergoing radiation treatments. It wasn't going to thrive in this spot no matter how much I watered it; it needed to be on the ground. I selfishly tried to make this poor plant live somewhere it constitutionally wasn't suited to, but it was never going to work for it. It ended up dying a crispy brown death there on my deck.

I clearly had some lessons to learn with plants. I had a lot to learn if I ever wanted to take care of another person, and I was curious about what I was missing in taking care of myself. I noticed that plants seemed to grow effortlessly when they were in the right environment and poorly when they were in the wrong one. I needed to know: Were there environments I did better or worse in? Was I like the red apple aptenia, or some other plant altogether?

These are important questions to ask because when you have a child, you want to know that your overall environment around you will also be supportive to your health and that of the ones you love. Bringing a child into a difficult life will only make it *more* difficult. You can be very selfish in evaluating this. If you aren't doing well, then you can't be your best for anyone else, either. This means looking at your body, behaviors, partner, and career; where you live; and the network of people who surround you, because this is the field that may later support the life of the baby.

The field is referred to as *kshetra* in Sanskrit. *Kshetra* is also used to refer to a place where a person may take a pilgrimage. Is getting created, being born, and living not the ultimate pilgrimage?

The field at a micro level is the cells, tissues, and organs surrounding the egg, as well as the uterus, and at a macro level it includes the broad environment surrounding the baby to come — all the way to the edge of the universe. First, we will focus on that which is most within our sphere of influence — our bodies. Later, we will focus on our environment and the people within it.

The Journey of an Egg

A fetus starts with a sperm and an egg. These are the two male and female seeds that come together to produce the baby. Earlier I mentioned that the fruit is the ovary of the strawberry plant, with all its little seeds that you can feel snap in your teeth as you chew them, but unlike the strawberry, a woman's ovary houses its eggs on the inside, so they are a little more difficult to see. In fact, you can really only see the eggs if you look through a microscope, which is kind of hard to do while a woman is alive and her ovaries are inside her.

Nature gives you your whole lot of eggs when you are in utero and then strategically divvies them out during your fertile years if they haven't already died off. The nutrients and hormonal levels during your life will affect the maturity, quality, growth, and death of these eggs. Significant events in a woman's life, as well as those of her partner and her parents, all play a role in her fertility. Nature thinks much more long-term than we humans do, and as life plays out, the actions of the past have an effect on the present and the future, though it is not impossible to change course once any patterns of imbalance become visible. Both you and nature affect your fertility.

Once a healthy follicle has shepherded an egg out of the ovary during ovulation, the egg ultimately needs to make its way toward the uterus, but it has to travel via a strange and indirect route. It is important to note that an egg can never move. It doesn't have a little tail the way a sperm does, so it can't swim through fluid or crawl alongside tissues. It is immobile. Any movement it makes is because something else moved it.

Adjacent to each ovary is a channel that provides a pathway into the uterus, the fallopian tube. What's fascinating about this connection between fallopian tube and ovary is that they are not physically attached. Rather, they are adjacent and have a little space between them. So, the egg that is destined to find its way into the uterus has to first cross through this little space, which is full of fluid. It is able to make this journey because the fallopian tube has fingerlike projections near the ovary, called *fimbriae*, which swell with blood around ovulation and start wiggling around in the fluid. It is through their movement that the newly ovulated egg is gently ushered through the fluid and into the fallopian tube, like a watery pinball game.

Once the egg makes it inside the fallopian tube, it needs a way to travel to the uterus, but as stated before, the egg cannot move itself, because it has no arms, legs, tail, or other appendages to move *with*. The egg instead gets help from the fallopian tube. Tiny hairlike structures called *cilia* on the inside cells start to carry the egg deeper into the tube, like a crowd-surfer at a concert. All the egg has to do is sit back, relax, and listen to the music while the hairs carry it down the pipeline.

It is here, inside the fallopian tube, that conception typically takes place. A sperm that has been ejaculated into a woman's vagina, squeezed through the small opening in the center of her cervix, and made it through the uterus just might also find its way into the fallopian tube containing the egg. This tube is where all the swimming sperms that have made it that far will compete with each other to be the first to penetrate the patiently waiting egg.

If a sperm is able to penetrate the egg, conception takes place, and the egg and sperm fuse together to form a zygote. A zygote is the first complete cell of the newly formed embryo, and the true seed of a unique individual. All other female and male seeds prior to this were incomplete, since both seeds are required for reproduction. The zygote is then delivered by those little cilia in the fallopian tube to the uterus, where it will attempt implantation into one of the walls. If that is successful, then the woman is pregnant. The process of gestation occurs and the zygote grows into more and more cells, becoming an increasingly complex organism in utero for approximately forty weeks (give or take), or until the mother's body goes into labor and the baby is born.

If conception does not take place, the hormone levels secreted by the egg to build up the uterine lining for implantation gradually decrease as the egg loses its vitality, and the uterine lining, along with the egg, blood, and any sperm left over, will be shed out during menstruation within a matter of days. Nature builds up tissues and breaks them down based on cues in the environment.

The Uterus

The uterus is the most direct and literal meaning behind the idea of the field in the Four Fertility Factors, because it's where a complete

human life implants and grows inside the amniotic sac with the umbilical cord and placenta. For a fetus, the uterus is ground zero of a larger
field set up to house its transition to the planet. It is an organ with
three major layers, each having a unique purpose. There is an epithelial
layer (sort of like a skin layer) and a muscle and vascular layer, and then
a layer of connective tissue. Possessing each of these parts, the uterus
has the ability to fill with blood and nutrients; to protect and lubricate
itself; and to grow, shrink, receive, or expel physical material.

Like all other organs, the uterus contains a hollow space inside the
body. Space is the container for all creation to occur. The uterus's space
can be quite vast and flexible. Because of all this openness, themes of
vulnerability and receptivity frequently come up when dealing with
the reproductive system, especially if there have been imbalances or
past traumas. You may have already heard that the word *hysteria*, derived from the ancient Greek root meaning "womb," was related to the
notion of a "wandering womb." Indeed, many complexities and much
mystery and drama are connected with this organ, but through studying her menstrual cycles, a woman can actually get a peek into her
overall health and begin to use the cycles as a guide. Each cycle tells the
story of how a woman lived her life in the month prior. The amount of
blood; its color and texture; the duration of the bleeding; the length of
time since the last period; the body swelling, cramps, headaches, mood
drops — these all demonstrate how a woman has balanced nature's
attributes, the gunas, and the wind currents, the vayus, in the previous
month. Paying attention to the details of your cycle will teach you a lot.

Many women want to know what a perfect period looks like, and
there is no specific answer. Because each egg and sperm will be slightly
different, in terms of the gunas they possess, no single idea of a perfect uterine condition for implantation exists. However, there are some
concepts that are universally helpful to know. Healthy tissues in the
mother's uterus are paramount. We know a tissue is healthy when it
is getting adequate blood flow and fluids, not too much or too little.
We know a tissue is healthy when it does not contain any blockages
of channels, such as inflammatory conditions or growths, like tumors,
cysts, or polyps. For flow to happen well, a channel must have space

inside it and be structurally intact and moderately pliable. Pain can sometimes be present when there is a blockage. Pain is a teacher we must listen to and study.

The uterus still does its work during the fertile years, even if a woman isn't getting pregnant. It practices and goes through the motions each month so that when it does come into that perfect space of conception, it will be healthy and ready to receive, grow, and gestate. It also continues so that a woman can learn from it how she is living her life.

The reproductive system is one of the last systems of the body to be prioritized when it comes to nourishment. Other essential physiological functions have more immediate importance to the maintenance of the life of the woman. Therefore, if the reproductive system is healthy, there's a good chance that the rest of the body is healthy, too. If imbalances exist, there may also be imbalances in other areas of the body.

The Important Role of Follicles

A woman's primary oocytes are stored inside follicles, so they are also part of the field for the egg. You may have heard of a follicle before because your hair grows out of follicles. There is a follicle for each egg in the ovary. They were joined together in the final processes of seed creation while your oocytes were being formed in utero. Similar to the way a hair follicle provides an incubating shell for the strand of hair growing out of it, an ovarian follicle provides a protective layer around the oocyte until it's fully manifested. If it's the seed destined to be released in that cycle, the follicle ultimately ushers the seed toward its exit from the ovary, kicks it out, and stays behind in the ovary to emit some progesterone, which thickens the lining of the uterus to nourish the seed if it becomes fertilized by male seed — sperm — so it can implant there. The follicle continues to support its seed for a while from afar but will die when its job is done — in a matter of weeks if pregnancy does not occur.

There is great interest in follicles because they provide a clue to how many primary oocytes a woman has left. Women undergoing medical fertility treatments will have a blood test done during a specific time of the month to see how many follicles are actively growing in that particular menstrual cycle. The blood test measures anti-Mullerian hormone (AMH), which is secreted by cells within the follicles when those follicles become activated for growth. Since you can't cut a woman open and see how many eggs she has left, the best guess is to estimate her number of follicles. Another way is to look at the ovaries with an ultrasound and see how many primary follicles are visible.

The authors of ancient Ayurvedic medical texts did not have microscopes and ultrasounds, though somehow they knew that men and women each contributed material in order for a child to develop. However, they were not able to see the intricate details of the woman's contribution to fertility and know something as specific as the fact that there are follicles forming a protective layer around an oocyte. Being able to look under a microscope has given us so much more tangible information about how humans are created. Today, we can look inside a woman, an ovary, or a follicle and visually verify what lies within at that moment in time. This is a great example of how modern technology has strengthened our understanding of the body.

At the same time, the ancient Ayurvedic scholars did know about the power of follicles on the exterior of the body, which is something that modern medicine is only starting to learn about today. In Ayurveda, the skin is not merely a passive layer of separation between our bodies and the outside world. It is a living tissue that has a two-way communication mechanism, and the follicles play an important role in this communication. First, there are nerve endings in the skin that inform us of sensations, and each hair follicle has a plexus of nerves that inform the brain about hairs that move. We can all feel that the skin excretes because we've all experienced sweating before, but what few people realize is that the skin also absorbs. Skin is permeable, and follicles play a key role because they represent a space through which liquid and other subtle matter can travel. In fact, there are studies showing that even caffeine applied to the skin will be detectable in the blood within twenty minutes. This mechanism is exploited in all topical medicines, such as patches and creams, but when you really think about it, it makes you realize that *everything* you put on your skin is likely to get into your bloodstream.

The reason it's important to think about skin here is because, like the follicles on the outside of your body, follicles in your ovaries are a type of channel for things to flow in and out of. Again, nature likes to repurpose formats where it can. The channel is first opened when the primary oocyte is developed in utero, and then it becomes activated when the follicle for that particular oocyte begins growing, only releasing the seed if it is the lucky one to be ovulated in a particular menstrual cycle. As with all channels, follicles can either be open and clear, or they can become clogged with toxins (internally or externally produced). Like getting clogged pores or acne on the surface of your skin, the follicles within your ovaries are also susceptible to clogging and blockages if they receive imbalanced nutrients because your metabolic health is suboptimal or because your doshas (bodily humors) are imbalanced. This is why it's critical to see the connection between your diet, your digestive health, and your reproductive functioning — and, for that matter, the outside of the body, the skin, too.

Water

As mentioned in the last chapter, water is one of the five elements. Water is the element specifically responsible for the action of lubrication and mixing. All the liquids in the body are essentially one body of water that changes its properties as it travels across the various membranes. Cells, nutrients, and hormones are transported inside these liquids.

Water is also what enables our sense of taste. When a person's mouth becomes dehydrated, the taste buds can get weakened. Therefore, water is also responsible for some of our ability to perceive our environment accurately.

Reading the Water

We need water. It helps other elements mix, but too much water — especially in a cold body — will dilute the body's power. Without adequate lubrication, we cannot taste our food fully and we cannot enjoy sex. On the other hand, an overly watery body is a sign of emotional attachment. Again, there is a perfect balance to be struck with all the elements — including water.

Many women think they are supposed to drink a certain amount of water — perhaps they've heard that doing so is good for them — but in reality, a woman must drink the amount needed for the environmental demands and the actions of *her* body. Water can be taken in too little and even too much quantity. I've had many clients who were actually weakening their digestive processes from drinking too much water. Checking out the color of one's urine is a good indicator of the level of hydration — the clearer, the more hydrated; and the more yellow/orange, the more dehydrated.

Water also affects body temperature. If we are more watery, it takes longer to change our body temperature. A body can be like the ocean or like the land. If like the ocean, it will heat and cool slowly, and if dry like the land, it will heat and cool more rapidly. This is worth considering because a woman's body temperature typically increases around the time of ovulation.

The temperature of the water consumed matters, too, because it affects metabolism and assimilation. Heat is necessary for metabolic power. A cold, wet body will have weak digestion.

In the case where a woman becomes pregnant, her body's capacity to hold water will increase dramatically, but until that happens, she needs only the amount that is good for it in its nonpregnant state. Too much water can begin to weaken her body's power. She must act according to the current biological demands of life, always.

The following chapter will help you identify whether your water element is balanced and also determine whether your other elements are balanced, or if adjustments can be made to allow your body to operate more optimally.

EXERCISE: HONORING THE PURPOSE OF THE REPRODUCTIVE SYSTEM

It is important to understand the purpose of sexual reproduction. Place your hand on your low belly, a few inches below your belly button, to feel the home of your reproductive organs. Even though you may have been enjoying sex for pleasure, love, or connection for many years, the purpose of sex, biologically speaking, is producing babies. Take a moment to honor the miracle that it is and your part in it.

This cognitive shift is key because your relationship with sex just got a whole lot more impactful. And, yes, you should still enjoy how pleasurable sex can be. Pleasure can be a wonderful side effect of sex.

Recap of the Four Fertility Factors

The reproductive system builds up when the conditions of the environment, life, and the body trigger such growth, and it will break down when the conditions are no longer supportive of such functions. For example, a woman's uterus grows to house a fetus, amniotic sac, placenta, and umbilical cord, as well as the water the baby grows inside of, but then it expels these things and shrinks back down after the baby is born. Similarly, her breasts develop and grow very large after childbirth and typically shrink back down once breastfeeding ceases. As menopause sets in, the ovaries shrink more each year. Organs, like muscles, grow and are maintained when they are getting energy and atrophy when they are not.

Most people understand that they came from Mom's egg and Dad's sperm joining forces, but few understand the intricacies of how this really happens and the history behind how the eggs and sperm came to be. Here, we will focus mostly on the woman's part of this reproductive equation, though it is important that both the male and female reproductive functioning be in tip-top shape and free from any block-ages, growths, or toxicity for optimum fertility. Since this is a book for women, we are focusing mostly on you.

You have a garden in your belly. Earth, water, and seeds are being held in a storage bin waiting to be released, planted, fertilized, and watered. Each organ of your reproductive system plays an important part in this garden, which was largely planted when you were still in your mother's womb. All your basic parts, cell types, and organs grew while you were inside your mother's belly from the genetic material your mom and dad both contributed, along with the nourishment your mom consumed from her environment while she was pregnant.

Like all your eggs, your reproductive organs were also gifted during this time, though they would not be used for their purpose until many years later. Each reproductive part in your pelvic area has its own unique role in this garden — the ovaries, uterus, vagina, cervix, fallo-pian tubes, and so on. In addition, some organs a little farther away from the pelvis — the breasts and the hypothalamus and the anterior pituitary gland in the brain — also have major contributing roles in reproductive functioning.

The reproductive system is affected by the whole body and also by the environment. Information, in the form of sounds, feelings, sights, tastes, and smells, travels via the sense organs and nerves to the brain and then from the brain via the nerves and hormones to organs of action in your body, including your reproductive system. This is why focusing only on your hormones for balance is limiting and study-ing mind-body health is so important; hormones are affected by the senses, thoughts, diet, and the doshas. The reproductive system is part of a larger whole, and it's pretty perceptive and efficient, as long as it hasn't been hindered or obstructed.

Having the working biology to create, house, and pop out a new life is a gigantic privilege — despite some of the discomforts of preg-nancy and the pain of labor. And even though your period may seem annoying at times, it's a useful cycle, and it actually comes with special powers you may have felt before, such as increased sense perceptions

at certain times of the month. It also gives you a peek into the quality of your blood, which helps you understand the rest of your body
and even your behaviors and actions. You can actually use your period
to your advantage — if you get to know it well. First, you must deepen
your knowledge of this part of yourself by studying how it works. Then
you can leverage its powers — and as a bonus, you make your body a
welcome home to live in.

Chapter 5

Discovering Your Type

According to Ayurveda, the first requirement for healing oneself
and others is a clear understanding of the three dosha.

— **VASANT LAD,** *Ayurveda: The Science of Self-Healing*

The reproductive organs are but one system in your whole body. Yes, it is the central system involved in making your body receptive to having a child, but it is affected greatly by the overall body — all the sense organs, tissues, and channels, along with metabolism — and your mental state. Your mental state is affected by your current environment, as well as past experience and memory (both mental and cellular). Your environment can have a direct impact on your biology, simply because you interact with it and it triggers responses in your body.

To determine what a particular body needs in a particular environment, it is important to look at the dominant dosha(s) for that person. Health is relative to the individual. Many women are not their healthiest because they are living the way they think is healthy for other people, rather than truly understanding what *they* need in order to be healthy. There is a difference, and until you see it, you won't know that one even exists. A woman must break the cycle of treating her body the way other women are treating their bodies — because her and their constitutions, life histories, and demands are very different. Even highly reputable scientific studies cannot be the top authority on an individual woman, because a woman is not an average, nor does research typically recognize that there are individual body types, not to mention the fact that science changes all the time, depending on the specific angle or agenda of those who commission or oversee it. As long as a woman thinks there are things that are universally healthy — such as eating a specific superfood, exercising a certain number of hours a week, or taking in the perfect amount of protein or carbohydrates according to some fad diet — then she doesn't truly know herself. Ayurveda is the science of getting to know oneself for real.

You can see when you look at very small children that they are different — one is very laid-back, another is more sensitive, and yet another is quicker to boss the others around. We each have a "way" about us. It's what makes life so interesting. Wouldn't it be so boring if we were all the same?

When I supervised the Infant Studies lab as an undergraduate psychology student, we would call these differences between individual babies *temperament*. Some people call these differences *energy* or *vibe*. In Ayurveda, we connect this psychological temperament with the physical characteristics and physiological functioning of the body. Energy and matter are interconnected. Nature makes us a certain way when we are conceived, and we spend our whole lives shifting further away from nature or returning back to it.

Are you ready to explore your nature? If yes, then start by taking the following quiz to begin to discover your doshic tendencies.

EXERCISE: DISCOVERING YOUR DOSHAS

Check the box next to the category that best represents your condition. Tally up the checks at the bottom of each column to get a sense of your dominant doshas.

DOSHA ASSESMENT

Body Composition Type

Skin	❏ Thick and cool; can get growths and skin tags	❏ Oily; reddens, gets rashes, or freckles easily	❏ Thin and delicate; tendency toward dryness or roughness
Hair	❏ Thick and plentiful	❏ Requires frequent washing due to oiliness; fine or medium thickness	❏ Frizzy or wild
TOTALS	____ **KAPHA**	____ **PITTA**	____ **VATA**

Excretion/Waste Type

Evacuation	❏ Solid and long stools; digestion can be slower	❏ Tendency toward looser stools; may be yellowish at times	❏ Irregular stools; may struggle to pass or have hard, dark feces
Urination	❏ Large volume of urine; can be cloudy	❏ Potential for burning or UTIs; urine may be yellow	❏ Frequent urination
Sweat	❏ Profuse sweating with intense exercise	❏ Constant sweating; can get smelly	❏ Minimal or no sweating
TOTALS	____ **KAPHA**	____ **PITTA**	____ **VATA**

Energy Type

Energy	❏ Slow-building, but steady and sustaining	❏ Intense; can suffer from burnout	❏ Prone to swings
Work habits	❏ Routine-oriented, slow, and thorough	❏ Ambitious and busy; influences others and is a doer	❏ Full of out-of-the-box ideas; tends to be unfocused
Sleep	❏ Can sleep any-time, anywhere	❏ Tires oneself out and crashes or stays up too late being busy	❏ Has difficulty getting to sleep or maintaining sleep
TOTALS	____ **KAPHA**	____ **PITTA**	____ **VATA**

Mental Tendencies Type

Temperament	❏ Calm and loyal; prone to attach-ment, addic-tion, sadness, grief, greed, stubbornness	❏ Sharply focused; a leader; prone to be in-tense, angry, frustrated, hypercritical, aggressive	❏ Broad think-ing, creative, changeable; prone to fear, doubt, anxiety, worry
Learning and memory	❏ Slower learner, but retains what is learned forever	❏ Quick learner with sharp focus and average memory	❏ Quick learner with poor focus and memory
TOTALS	____ **KAPHA**	____ **PITTA**	____ **VATA**

Menstrual Patterns Type

Cycle length	❏ Slow cycles (>28 days)	❏ Frequent (<28 days) or perfectly on-time cycles	❏ Disrupted or absent cycles (sometimes <28 days and sometimes >28 days)
Menstrual bleeding	❏ Bleeding for many days, in moderate amounts, possibly with mucus or membranes	❏ Heavy bleeding or spotting between periods	❏ Scanty, dry, brown, or black blood, or bleeding for a short duration or not at all
TOTALS	____ **KAPHA**	____ **PITTA**	____ **VATA**

Which dosha do you think is most dominant in your system, according to this test? And is the menstrual type the same as the rest of you? You may actually find that more than one dosha is high, and that different doshas are out of balance in different parts of the body — but typically one will emerge above the others. This can also change seasonally. Keep this in mind as you read further. You may begin to see the signs of the doshas in your body more clearly as we go.

Disease Progression and Reversal

Remember from earlier in the book that a dosha is something that can go out of balance? You'll recall that there are three — vata, pitta, and kapha. In nature, they are the movement, transformation, and protection, respectively. In the body, we could summarize them by saying they are air, blood, and mucus. We need all three doshas, but in balanced amounts. However, we tend to have higher amounts of some than others.

According to Ayurveda, imbalanced doshas are found at the root of all diseases. If left unchecked, they accumulate, move, spread, and then take over weakened tissues of the body, which is when symptoms occur. This is how diseases form. Understanding the first signs of imbalanced doshas — along with the ways in which a dosha may have moved through a body, and why — is a key to understanding how a disease started and how to reverse it before it becomes a manifested or progressed disease.

Stages of Disease in Ayurveda

Disease happens in stages. Individuals who have good body awareness are likely to feel that there is an issue in the beginning stages, while those who do not have much body awareness may not determine that a disease process is at work until later stages, until symptoms have emerged and are possibly already causing complications. It turns out that being healthy requires body awareness. This is one of the reasons why many people who are into yoga, meditation, or fitness are very interested in Ayurveda. It works when you pay attention to your body, and it doesn't work when you ignore your body. If you pay attention to your body, you can detect and treat imbalances and diseases early.

The home site of vata (space + air) is the colon, so individuals with accumulating vata may experience constipation or dry, hard stools. Pitta's (fire + water) home site is in the small intestine because that's where bile and pancreatic and other transformative gastric juices converge for processing food into a substance that is usable by the body, so high pitta may show up as heartburn an hour or two after a meal, or in loose, burning stools or diarrhea. Pitta also shows up a lot in the liver, spleen, blood, and sweat. Kapha's (water + earth) home sites include the upper part of the stomach, lungs, mucous membranes, and joints. Accumulating kapha, being wet earth, manifests as a sense of wetness, heaviness, or congestion in these areas, sometimes even accompanied by nausea.

Vata may start as gas or bloating but then might turn into dehydration and constipation, later into muscle spasms and popping and cracking joints, and finally into some dry or degenerated tissue. (Examples include dry, rough external skin if it is getting an excess of vata energy; vaginal dryness or dry sinus if mucosal skin in those areas is getting too much vata energy; or memory issues if the brain is getting increased vata energy due to lack of sleep, too much worrying, a high-vata diet, or being blocked from receiving vital fluids.)

Pitta may start as a burning sensation in the belly, which then might spread to other parts of the body and finally turn into inflammation or redness appearing in a tissue. (Examples include red rashes or acne on the external skin and issues of heavy bleeding or even overproduction of red blood cells; issues with the liver, spleen, and kidneys are also common, as these organs are filtering blood, which can contain the excess pitta.)

Kapha may start as a sense of fullness or heaviness in the chest or abdomen but then might turn into swelling; frequent urination; or slimy, leaky parts, later to manifest as metabolic issues, clogging, or tissue overgrowth due to the dulling of the fire element. (Examples include wet asthma; weight gain; high cholesterol; or tumors, cysts, and skin tags.)

Modern medicine is typically focused on the later stages of disease. Unfortunately, once you get past certain points, it is a little harder to rebalance a body naturally. Late-stage disease conditions include cancer that has metastasized and diabetes that has started to cause vision problems or wound-healing issues.

Furthermore, Ayurveda categorizes symptoms in two different ways: warning signs and symptoms. The first category is a *purvarupa*, or a premonitory symptom, meaning that you can sense that something is off, but it hasn't necessarily turned into something perceived as bad for the body yet. Purvarupas tell you that something bad may be on its way. For example, have you ever gotten the sense that you are extremely fatigued, and then that evening you feel a fever or a cold come on?

A *rupa*, on the other hand, is an actual symptom of illness. You may have a feeling that your sinuses are dry or burning (purvarupa), and the next day you wake up with a stuffy nose. This is an example of vata aggravating your sinuses, creating inflammation (pitta) and possibly causing excess mucus (kapha) to be sent to the sinuses to help heal the tissues.

In my sinus example above, the rupa would be a congested or runny nose. It's a sensation that there is a true imbalance and that the body is trying to heal it. Rupas get a bad rap because they do not feel good, but oftentimes they are actions the body is taking to get us back to homeostasis, and if we try to interfere with them, we can make them worse. The rupa itself isn't the problem, because it was actually caused by something else — and Ayurveda is the art and science of getting at the "something else."

I remember sleeping in a large dorm room full of women when I was staying in an ashram in India, and there were ceiling fans above our heads to keep us cool while we were sleeping. Because I know that too much wind dries my sinuses out, I covered my mosquito net above my face with a towel to block the air when I went to bed. I was one of the only women in the dorm who did not get a stuffy nose during my stay at the ashram! People sometimes have a hard time understanding that they can be making a cold worse by taking a decongestant if the root cause is dryness from too much air/vata. Mucus shows up on the scene to protect tissues from the wind. Similarly, inflammation wouldn't necessarily go away if you dry out the mucus. Instead, you would just be making it even more sensitive and reactive with a medicine that acts as a drying agent.

Sometimes we aren't getting sick due to a bug — sometimes we are getting sick because we are missing something in our environment and not adjusting our own behaviors accordingly. Bugs get the better of us when our immune system is at its weakest. The immune system gets weak when sensory processing is impaired or when our minds make poor choices.

How Doshas Contribute to Disease

When a dosha accumulates and becomes aggravated, it can leave its home site; enter into the bloodstream, lymph, or other bodily channels; and be transported to areas of the body that are (1) taking some sort of action and are using energy/nourishment, or (2) simply receiving energy/ nourishment due to gravity. If there is a weakness in any of the tissues along the way — whether it is your skin, muscle, fat, brain, bones, marrow, or reproductive organs — that weakened tissue may also begin to absorb the imbalanced dosha, which will then interfere with the quality of that local tissue. This is how disease manifests and spreads.

This is how reactive digestion can transfer to the skin and cause acne. This is how constipation can turn into the wasting away of your fat, muscle, or skin. This is also how the slimy nature of excess mucus — which contains sugars, lipids, and proteins — can later contribute to the development of cysts, tumors, and other abnormal tissue growths. The body is a master at converting materials into different forms when it has a reason to.

How Imbalances Progress

There are several possible reasons why an individual may not have body awareness and therefore allow a disease to progress. The first is referred to as *asatmendriyartha samyoga*, a misuse of the senses, where someone is misperceiving the environment due to a sensory imbalance. A sensory detail is missed or interpreted incorrectly, as in the preceding case with the stuffy noses in the ashram dorm.

The second cause of disease is referred to as *kala parinama*, where a person is not respecting that there are natural changes produced by the passage of time. The body undergoes changes as the environment shifts during the course of a day or seasonally; this is homeostasis at work. In addition, bodies have certain patterns that develop as life progresses. If we fail to observe these natural patterns, or if we try to outsmart or avoid them in any way, then we may contribute to imbalances. It is always best to live in harmony with time. Not following the circadian rhythm has been linked to so many general health issues, and for women of the fertile years, that includes irregular and longer menstrual cycles.

Ayurveda is a science of longevity, and respecting and honoring the seasons of life and time is part of allowing the cells to operate optimally. For example, pitta naturally builds in summer, so if by the end of the summer, a person has been favoring too many pitta-aggravating foods, such as salty, sour, pungent foods or an excess of meat, then this person may end up with inflammatory issues, rashes, or other pitta symptoms. We can assume that perhaps the individual was not respecting the need for more cooling sensory input and foods in summer, and detoxification may be necessary.

The last cause of disease is *prajnaparadha*, a misuse of the intellect, whereby we may simply be using irrelevant conditioning and faulty logic to make decisions or conclusions, and it's these poor decisions that lead to actions that are causing disease. Our logic and decision-making are programmed from past experience, and if we do not challenge these patterns, then we will find they are outdated — not *if* but *when* the environment around us changes. Conditioning can also override sensory input. These are the ways we actually harm *ourselves*.

The most effective way to remove an illness is *nidana parivargana* — to remove the cause of the illness — and the body will heal itself. However, why does this seem so difficult for all of us to do? Why the heck do we seem attached to foods, experiences, lifestyles, and even people that are not healthy for us? Why do we build cities where there is no water flowing and then redirect a river to keep it operating, rather than simply living near the water?

We often cannot determine the cause because it does not match our logic, or because we are simply not paying attention to it. We may be distracted by our thoughts, our environment, higher-priority desires, or some severe pain that we're avoiding. Can we really trust ourselves? Since 55 percent of Americans regularly take prescription medications — four, on average — some of which can alter a person's perception of the environment, it could be argued that more than half of us cannot trust our own minds.

Even when one pays keen attention and detects a subtle problem, it can be easy to get used to a minor imbalance of the body and then stop paying attention to it, but these imbalances are adding up over time. A small ongoing imbalance is like the constant drip from a leaky faucet that in time will fill up a bucket, and after that a bathtub, and then drip down to the neighbor's apartment below — then the mold starts to grow everywhere. Somehow we've become tolerant of the drip and have stopped paying attention to its damaging potential.

In summary, Ayurveda teaches that people obtain diseases during their lifetime because some crime against nature has been repeatedly committed. Sure, there are environmental toxins, too, but it's up to you to perceive them and then to make choices to reduce their levels in your system or move away from them. I know this isn't easy to hear, especially if you feel you've come in contact with some environmental toxicity, but your health always depends on your ability to balance your body in an environment.

Balancing your body means having your doshas in equilibrium, healthy tissues, a regular appetite, and an intellect and sensory processing that can be trusted. So if you have detected environmental toxins, you will be wise not to ignore them but rather to take action to oppose the qualities of the toxins. If there's a small fire on your kitchen stove, it may be safe enough to grab the fire extinguisher and put it out yourself, but if the whole room has already gone up in flames, get the heck out, call 911, and let the experts at the fire department put it out. One you can handle on your own, and the other requires much more help.

Luckily, nature is somewhat forgiving. It allows us to commit a mistake or two. If we quickly make choices that are based on wholeness again, then the body has the ability to be a self-correcting system. However, if we continue on our faulty path, our choices start to add up and the disease process progresses. Suddenly bodily channels become inflamed, blocked, or degenerated, and then we need further help to rebalance. Sometimes a disease process goes so far that it causes additional complications, and unfortunately, some diseases progress so far that there is no cure.

This is why it's always best to try to address early-stage disease. The longer an imbalance goes on or the more it intensifies, the more it will progress. Nature will reward you for paying attention early, so try your best.

Understanding Cravings

One of my clients was in the process of breaking up with someone, and she kept gravitating toward the artwork of Georgia O'Keeffe — not the lush, flowery paintings of hers but the ones that had lots of desert scenes and skulls in them. She was craving a little bit of death and breaking-down, so indulging in these destructive forms was actually beautiful to me. She was channeling Shiva and Kali, archetypes of destruction.

We get inspirations and cravings for different energies in our lives sometimes. There is one challenge with a craving: it's difficult to know if it's harmful or beneficial. Cravings can arise out of need or can be attachments to something we are used to, and it's hard to know the difference. This is where Ayurveda and yoga come in, specifically the act of denying oneself something, as in the practice of cutting off sensory input or abstaining from food, because it is in this denying that we can see how we really feel without it. If we can get into a clear and present state while we are in self-denial, then we can see what we truly need.

This particular client was juicy and robust. She had stable routines and was very stuck in her life. She wasn't happy with her job, and she was having metabolic issues and difficulty getting pregnant. I felt this desire for a little bit of destruction could very well be a healthy craving for her. If instead of being juicy and robust, she had been suffering from dryness and emaciation or began isolating herself from others, then I possibly would have recommended she find some art of a jungle river with turtles swimming in it.

Ayurveda is all about artfully driving our lives as ongoing science experiments. We do tests, learn something, refine our understanding, and repeat the process. In every moment, we are all doing the best we can. If we start craving these same destruction-inspiring Georgia O'Keeffe images or feel an urge to head out to the desert to go to Burning Man while suffering from emaciation, insomnia, and constipation — signs of vata imbalance — then we can probably guess that this is a craving for what we are used to, rather than what we need in this moment.

Metabolic Factors in Health and Disease

A disease is created either because the doshas alone are imbalanced or because they are imbalanced and a second layer of pathology is also wreaking havoc on the body: an imbalanced metabolism. When the body's digestive and metabolic fire, *agni*, is not balanced, it will not digest your food or experiences well, and the poorly processed particles in the body form a type of toxic sludge, called *ama*. You may be familiar with plaque, such as on the teeth, in the arteries, or even in the brain. Ayurveda would refer to such plaques and the tartar on the teeth as ama. It gets into your body the same way properly digested food does, except it's improperly digested, unable to be used by the body, and starts to interfere with normal physiological processes and intercellular transport. It comes in various forms, depending on the foods you ate and the quality of your digestive juices, enzymes, and the like. You may notice it as a coating on the tongue at times. (Have you ever looked at your tongue in the mirror when you first wake up? If you see something coating it, that's ama.)

Ama can clog and block the vital channels of the body and disrupt the flow of liquids, solids, and air from passing through normally. When clogging occurs, it ultimately causes decay, disease, or degeneration on the would-be receiving end of the tube with the blockage, and the backup pressure from the blockage then disrupts the normal flow patterns of other channels. Having clear bodily channels is how nutrients, along with mental and sensory experiences, reach the places where they are needed. Not having ama is the key to clear bodily channels, and having balanced agni is critical to preventing ama from forming.

Agni is actually the name of a fire god in ancient Vedic literature from India. Agni is fire, and fire is the desire to process and assimilate food and new experiences via sensory input. Agni goes even beyond digestion; it also governs your cellular fire and metabolism. In addition to digestive agni, an agni for each tissue of the body — plasma, blood, muscle, fat, bone, marrow, and so on — including reproductive tissue, is present. It is fueled by hunger and deep purpose. The main, ruling agni type of the body is that of the upper digestive system, so the gut is the best place to start trying to correct imbalances. The rest of the self learns and takes cues from it.

When your agni is low, you don't feel the need to eat much, and if you do eat, you want to consume foods that will boost your agni. Since agni governs your ability to digest your food and adequately assimilate the nutrients in it, it is your key to preventing your body from getting all clogged up with toxic sludge.

Conversely, if your agni is too strong, you will be ravenously hungry most of the time, possibly to the point where you will get heartburn if you don't eat nourishing foods that lubricate you and cool you down. Without eating to satisfy the flame of your hunger fire, you may be causing gastric juices to burn the lining of your digestive organs. In this case, it's critical that you dampen your agni with cooling foods and slow, restorative activities.

You may also have mixed agni, where sometimes it's weak and sometimes it's strong. This is common for people who lack solid routines in their lives, including those who get out of sync with the circadian rhythms due to irregular work or sleeping patterns, as well as individuals going through life transitions like a breakup, job change, or move. The key to having regular agni is to spend your time aligning your basic routines of eating, sleeping, exercising, and working with the cycles of nature. If you overeat or eat at the wrong times (when agni is not strong, for example, or too frequently), food may not be processed adequately, and the large, unprocessed molecules of food (ama) can begin to clog up the digestive tract or cause a reaction — or worse, they can make their way into the blood, lymph, and other tissues to cause disease if the gut wall is compromised. You want balanced agni to have a healthy body.

Many women are told by their medical doctors that a reproductive-health issue is due to a metabolic disorder, but few women truly understand what this means. There are three types of metabolic disorders according to Ayurveda:

- The first type is a **slow metabolism**. It typically means the woman has low agni and is eating too much or too frequently or she is indulging in more dense, heavy, wet, or cooling foods than her body really needs. This dulling of agni can result in a woman even losing some of her energy and passion for life.

- The second type is a **sharp metabolism**, which can cause a person to be very hungry and put on weight or burn a body out and damage tissues. Balancing a high metabolism requires cooling down so that the body does not demand so much and eating foods that are cooling and sustaining.
- The third type is an **erratic metabolism**. In this case, sometimes it's high and sometimes it's low. The person lacks routine and self-discipline. Once the lifestyle behaviors are regulated, then agni will balance out to a level that is more predictable.

Each body has a different nourishment requirement for its lifestyle, so unlike in modern medicine, an Ayurvedic practitioner likely won't tell you that you need some magic number for your weight or body mass index (BMI). Instead, the focus is on helping you continuously develop good-quality bodily tissues that allow you to meet the demands of the life you love to live, in the environment where you are. Balancing your agni helps with this. There's no single medical test you can take to figure out if your agni is balanced, but you can observe and feel your body to learn about it.

When agni is imbalanced in the digestive tract and ama (the yucky sludge) forms, this toxic material can be delivered to the organs involved in a particular bodily function or system. Such toxins clog or inflame, blocking cellular intelligence and the flow of nutrients through microchannels of the body, causing abnormalities in tissues. This is one way your digestion can interfere with your reproductive system. Therefore, when you're studying your reproductive health, it's important to also study the digestive condition.

I had a client once who had such sharp agni that eating three meals a day, plus snacks, was not nearly enough for her. Her stomach was burning all the time because she couldn't keep up with the demands of her agni, and her gastric juices, in the absence of the right kind of diet to keep them busy, were irritating the lining of her digestive organs. She needed to either reduce her activity level dramatically to decrease the demands of her body or start eating foods that could counterbalance the sharp agni, such as creamy, sweet, cooling foods. In one month, we were able to rebalance her system with a few small diet modifications, herbs, a little less activity, and some restorative yoga.

Many people can see evidence of rebalancing in one month, though healing often takes many more months, depending on how far an imbalance has progressed. It's very easy for humans to fall back into old patterns when the same environmental triggers still exist around them, so healing must be viewed as a practice that takes a bit of time. Healing requires the most brutal, honest look at oneself. A common complaint about conventional medicine is that it does not help patients get at the root cause of disease, but the same thing can happen with Ayurveda if people do not look deeply into themselves.

Hunger is a good signal of agni. It is important to understand that hunger is not the same as appetite. Many times we eat due to routine and cravings — not when we feel the actual growling, burning sensation that comes with true hunger. It can be difficult to discern the difference. I frequently work with clients who have no sense of true hunger. For some, this is because they are keeping such regular eating routines that they never allow themselves a chance to experience it, while others have no true hunger because they ignored it for so long that the body got used to not signaling it.

Fasting is a practice that helps an individual understand the difference between appetite and hunger. At first during a fasting phase, hunger increases, and then after an extended period of time the agni becomes weakened. This is also one reason why fasting should not be practiced indefinitely. It is a form of medicine and should be treated as such with methodical practice, and in some cases with guidance. If hunger has become reduced, then a woman may use agni-promoting spices in the kitchen, such as ginger, different types of pepper, and cinnamon, as well as salt, lime, and vinegar, or she may start exercising more to bring it back to life.

Proper nourishment and metabolism, plus a favorable environment, are the keys to tissues developing properly. Balanced agni is key to proper metabolism and digestion, and preventing the clogging substance, ama. Your doshas *can* get out of balance even if your agni is balanced and you don't have any ama clogging the channels of your body, but doshic imbalances without ama are generally much less complicated to rebalance. First a person has to remove the ama, and then the doshas can be rebalanced. Trying to rebalance doshas without first clearing the ama means they will still flow irregularly through the body and cause disease. If a dam blocks a river, then the water is redirected.

Learning about your metabolic type can help you balance your body, your diet, and even your energy.

Which type of agni do you think you have?

AGNI TYPES

	BALANCED	WEAK	SHARP	IRREGULAR/ MIXED
SIGNS	Hunger for 2–4 meals or snacks per day, especially around midday, depending on energy output. Daily bowel movements (ideally in the morning) with no digestive issues.	Not much hunger even when skipping meals. Sluggish/slow digestion with a sense of fullness. Possible diarrhea or constipation.	Strong hunger and need to eat frequently. Experience of either burning in the upper GI tract or weight gain. Frequent bowel movements.	Alternation between weak and sharp agni. See previous columns.

Many factors affect agni, and symptoms of low agni will differ from individual to individual. With balanced agni, people will likely have stronger immunity and can then tolerate a broader mix of foods. Agni that is weak or imbalanced cannot process certain foods well, especially when eaten in larger quantities. As stated earlier, imbalances in your body can be either with or without that toxic sludge, ama. As you study your body more through the exercises provided in this book, I hope you begin to learn about your dominant doshas and whether you have any ama in your body. Later, you'll see some ways to balance these out.

The Connection between Overall Health and Reproductive Health

A healthy reproductive tract is needed for fertility, as is an overall healthy body. As with all other parts of the body, here communication of information takes place via electrochemical activity traveling through nerves, and nutrients are delivered via blood and other fluids. Any imbalances arising locally or transferred to other vital areas involved in the reproductive processes can block a healthy menstrual cycle. To contribute to the health of her seed, a woman must look at both her reproductive health and her overall health.

A healthy reproductive system is created the same way other healthy tissues are created in the body: through the balancing of the three doshas and your metabolic power, mind, and sensory processing. Health means that appropriate energy and resources are directed to the areas of the body responsible for generating the tissues needed for sustaining life in a certain environment. If energy is flowing and nutrients are appropriate, healthy growth can occur. However, if there are any blockages or damage in the channels leading to these organs, then a woman may experience insufficient tissue growth or malformations. Likewise, with too much energy and nutrients going to these organs, certain abnormal growth conditions can occur, such as cysts and tumors. All such imbalances can block a healthy menstrual cycle, the process that enables your fertility. Imbalances of the elements have a unique presentation in the reproductive system due to the special tissue types present and the frequency of change that the system undergoes.

A woman who has a major health issue in one system of the body can have problems in her reproductive area as well. When the body tries to heal an illness, it steals energy and resources from other areas, and sometimes it can kick its own defensive mechanisms into overdrive, which can confuse hormonal signals and information transfer. It is also possible for a woman to be completely healthy in other parts of her body and experience imbalances limited to the reproductive tract due to its unique physiology. No two women's bodies are the same.

As I've mentioned before, you want to be as healthy as possible when you conceive, and you want this health that you achieve to be something that you know how to get back to for the rest of your life, too. This is important, because when a child is conceived, it happens because there was the perfect environment present for it to succeed. Nature asks only that you be your true self, and in your constant commitment to this state of being, you will inherently be the best mother you can be.

Chapter 6

Engaging the Heart

You are the instrument in the hands of the Divine.

— RAMA JYOTI VERNON,
Yoga: The Practice of Myth and Sacred Geometry

A seed signifies the beginning of something — a plant, a human life, an idea. Within it lives the instructions and basic materials for an organism. But at the same time that a seed is a beginning, it is also an end. It represents a decision — a point in time when symmetry has been broken, a design is created, a code is written, and the whole thing is packaged up in a cute little box to get delivered somewhere later. When you make a decision to have unprotected sex, especially when you are fertile, you might get a chance to open up that box. Plant your seeds wisely; they will grow when the environment is right.

Understanding how seeds play a part in your fertility requires that we focus more broadly than simply considering the eggs you may have inside your ovaries — we must look to the whole you, plus your partner and your parents, as well as your environment and previous life experiences. But while these other actors and actions of the past all have a role in the creation of a child, you are not merely a bystander in the process. You are a designer, a priestess, and a muse. Through your own inspiration, you in turn inspire, and then you see what the universe does with this energy.

Invoking the Elements

The five elements are the basic building blocks of all matter in the universe, including the parts of your body, a baby, the food that nourishes you both, and the environment that provides support and excitement. Each element is important in fertility. To call these elements into yourself, you will do so by curating your environment. When you sense the elements around you, they will grow within you. The opposite is also true: once these elements are within you, you will also start to find them in other places.

Space

Space is the first and most important element to invoke in your creative process. Without space, there is no room for anything new to manifest. When a space opens up, it creates a vacuum for energy and matter to penetrate. The uterus has a space in the middle of it, which shrinks as the lining fills with blood and fluids as the menstrual cycle progresses after ovulation. Other spaces exist — in the vagina, in the center of the cervix, inside the fallopian tubes, between the fallopian tube and ovary, and even inside the follicle, which houses the female seed, or oocyte. These spaces are channels. In a healthy body, these channels are all unobstructed and energy can flow through them.

Space also exists between you and your partner. Though the emotional connection you have can feel binding at times, you will want to always keep a little bit of space between the two of you. This doesn't mean ignoring one another. It simply means that you observe your grasping and your attachments — both of these emotions, if too strong, will close the space. Your partner is a unique individual, with his own life and challenges. In order for a baby to enter your life, there must be some room for it. Space may create more desire at times, like anyone in a long-distance relationship can tell you, but when there is too much space, it can also kill desire — especially if this goes on for a long time. These two examples demonstrate the power of this element.

Air

You can't see air, but you can see what it moves. Air is responsible for the movement of fluids, hormones, seeds, blood, and so forth in the menstrual cycle and conception. Air is behind the electrochemical activity of the nerves and the pumping of blood through veins and arteries to the ovaries, uterus, and vagina. When the wind blows, you can feel it move the hairs on your head and sometimes, as I pointed out in chapter 3, even the tiny hairs on your arms. Such movements are happening inside you, too. If you could peek into a living fallopian tube, you would see the air element moving the water and little cilia inside, like blades of seagrass on the ocean floor.

Movement is necessary for life. The dramas we experience are our reactions and resistances to movement. We must be open to change if we want something new to happen. Therefore air challenges our ability to surrender.

Fire

Fire makes transformation possible. It makes us hungry, and it transforms nutrients into the tissues of our bodies. In the reproductive tract, fire is the blood and body heat necessary for ovulation to happen. It is in the desire for lovemaking that many women experience around ovulation, when they are "in heat."

Your desire for your partner is a power in your fertility process. Your arousal is paramount. Women are the temptresses of passion and the mistresses of seduction. There is a reason why passionate love is represented by red — it moves the blood. All acts that get you in the mood bring the fire element. Many women love to dance or wear lingerie, for example, to stimulate their inner temptress and the desire of their partner. You don't have to master the *Kama-sutra*, but even the ancient medical texts of Ayurveda talk about how a woman who enthralls her lover's senses is the best aphrodisiac for a man. A woman should first inspire herself, and then she will inspire her partner. At the end of the day, creating a baby is a passionate, animalistic process, so let loose and enjoy the ride.

Agni: Your Body's Fire God

Just like the digestive system, each of the tissues and individual cells has its own form of agni, or metabolic fire, which represents the body's ability to fully process what it has ingested, whether it is food, bits of information, or sensory input. The blood has a form of agni. The muscle has it, too, as do fat, bone, marrow, nerves, lymph, and your reproductive tissues. Even the little cells inside you that are shepherding new people into the world have agni. Remember, agni is a passionate hunger and desire, and the agni of your reproductive system, like other types, can be too strong or too weak.

Water

Water brings love into the reproductive process. Hormones are transported in water, and water lubricates the vagina for sexual intercourse. A baby needs water to develop in. Because water lubricates, it allows rapid growth and change to occur with less discomfort, so next time you feel like complaining about water weight, make sure to note that it's possibly protecting you from or enabling transformative processes inside you.

Water also provides a solution in which other elements can mix. Sperm is delivered through semen, which is a fluid. This fluid preserves the sperm, provides it nourishment, and ultimately allows it to reach the ovum.

Water can be still, or water can have lots of movement. If you lie in a sensory-deprivation tank, you will not feel the water once it becomes still. You will feel only your body floating in it. However, if there were suddenly waves in this water, you would feel the movement. Water is subtle but can also be very powerful. It provides just the right amount of resistance to keep the ocean cooler than the air around it in summer and warmer than the air in winter.

The sense of taste is associated with the water element. When the tongue is dry, the ability to taste is affected. Similarly, when a woman's vagina is dry, her taste for the pleasure of her partner's body is also weakened. The body must be adequately juicy for fertility. You are encouraged to savor your partner, and you need liquid to do that.

On the other hand, you can have too much water. As I mentioned before, people often become obsessed with drinking water because they heard it's good to drink a certain amount. I've worked with many clients who were in fact drinking way too much water, so that they were actually weakening their digestive enzymes and thus their main digestive agni. When this happens, the metabolism suffers and toxins can be created. In addition, when the main digestive agni gets compromised, it can compromise *all* the other agnis of the body. Had these people learned to trust their sense of thirst and understand how to read their excretions, rather than merely following some one-size fits all guideline or advice they heard along the way, they would have saved their agni. However, we know how this happens — sometimes we don't trust ourselves as much as we trust some other authority.

So we are a bit like plants — we need to be watered, but we need the right amount of water at the right times. And we need to learn to read our unique bodies and needs, rather than always do what we heard was healthy. Following advice blindly gets us only so far. Following the lead of the body...now that is perfectly juicy. If you are really tuned in and also have a good understanding of your health history, you can more expertly read your own body.

Earth

Earth comes from the food we eat, just as the food we eat comes from the earth. A woman will often feel the desire to eat more when she is pregnant and even during ovulation and just before her period, when the uterine lining is thickening; the earth element is needed to build bodies and tissues. Earth is in the physical structure of a human body, including in all reproductive organs. This element is present in women in a very individual way: some women have thick, luscious thighs and rounded buttocks, and others are leaner and lithe. We are not all meant to look the same, just as the baby for you is not the same as the baby for the woman next door.

Women who are craving more earth don't always have to eat more to get it. You can go for a hike in nature around big, sturdy trees and boulders to stimulate the earth energy within you. When the outdoors isn't an option, a nice houseplant can do the trick. On the other hand, if you are feeling too heavy and too earthy, it might be time to free yourself of some of the earth with lightening therapy, referred to in Sanskrit as *langhana*, such as fasting, cleansing, or exercising.

You are here on Earth, but right now, your future child is not. That child is in a different dimension. However, if you want that child to come to Earth, then you must do what creates matter. You need space for a baby — a place for movement, fire, water, and earth — and the right amount of space. You know it's the right amount because you feel alive and excited.

If you really want a child, do not grasp for a child. It's not the desire for a baby that makes a baby; it's the desire for sex. Also, even if you are longing for one, I don't recommend any of the numerous things that women do to sublimate their desire for a child — getting a pet, dating a much younger person, or becoming the mother to your family or everyone you work with — because it puts the energy you will need later for the baby elsewhere. Rather, create space and move your body like wild women have done for ages. If this creates fire with your partner, then perhaps the elements may come together to fuel creation of the baby.

Get flexible. Align with wonder. Find your passion. Be challenged. Surrender. Observe. Keep your creative spirit alive.

The Power of Rituals

It is essential for you to build poignant rituals into your everyday life as you prepare for getting pregnant, especially if you are like most modern people and feel overwhelmed by chaos. It's helpful to set up visual cues in your environment to inspire these effects. Otherwise, the void will get filled with things that are distracting and don't really make your heart sing. I recommend that if you are truly seeking a blessing from the universe, whether it is a child, a new job, a home, or anything else, you should set up an altar in your home. Not only can you freak your partner out by appearing to be a witch, but you can also set yourself up for a daily reminder of the dreams you are building. From now on, you may choose to establish a daily meditation practice in this spot. Here's how to create your space.

EXERCISE: CREATING SPACE FOR RITUALS

Find the Right Spot

Walk around your home and get a feel for all the rooms. Select one where you can be alone or where you spend a lot of time daily.

Next, look for the right spot in that room where you can place an altar for your regular inspiration, typically against a wall, on a windowsill, or on a desk or table. If your room is large enough, it can also be in the center. You need to see it regularly.

Create an Altar

Select a piece of furniture or even a windowsill that you can place some meaningful objects on. If you need a piece of furniture you don't have, your homework is to get creative and obtain one within seven days. You may choose to instead spread objects throughout the room — or throughout your house, for that matter — but the same principles will apply.

Collect Meaningful Objects

Elemental balancing: Find objects representing the elements you need more of, and place them on your altar.

> Space — objects that help you feel free and spacious, or items related to music
>
> Air — objects that represent movement and the sense of touch
>
> Fire — objects that represent your passion and make you feel warm inside
>
> Water — objects that feel cooling and fluid
>
> Earth — objects that are grounding, calming, and cooling

Personal inspirations: You may have an object that represents your fertility journey or inspires your sensual, feminine side. It may be something that you made, a token from a spiritual journey, or perhaps something you came across while on a vacation somewhere. Maybe it was a gift. Whatever it is, it should call forth the kind of energy you want to have with you on this journey. It's completely up to you.

Offer Blessings and Set Intentions

After the altar is complete, set aside a few minutes to bless it and commit to your intentions. Sit comfortably in the space. Take a few breaths, feeling the spine in the back of your body. Scan your whole creation with your peripheral vision. Then, look at each of the objects you have added. Remind yourself of your intentions in setting up this space. Sit for at least five minutes and meditate on it.

As you learn more about your constitutional type in the following chapters, you may want to add more of certain balancing elements to your ritual space. But first, let's delve into sound as a creative practice.

EXERCISE: EXPLORING PRIMORDIAL SOUND

Sound is the subtler form of the space element. It is connected to both the ear and the larynx (voice box). The ear senses sound, and the larynx creates sound. The practice of chanting or singing can be a powerful tool in tapping into the creative energy of nature. Your voice is pleasant music to the lover who will get you pregnant.

Simply chanting *om* is a way to explore the subtle element of sound. *Om* is a seed syllable used in mantras and has a deep connection to cycles of life: the opening of the mouth is birth, the sustaining of the *om* is life, and the closing of the mouth is death.

Another way to experiment is with your own intuitive sound that arises out of the silence when you sit quietly. To try this latter approach, sit in your ritual space or a quiet room (alone if you prefer) and just begin chanting long, sustained vowel sounds. Close your eyes and start with *A*, then *E, I, O, U*. Notice which sounds you like the most and return to them. Feel the vibration of the sound in your body. Scan the chest, head, throat, and even the deep core and pelvis as the sound vibrates through your body.

Explore a range of sound. Do not worry about what it sounds like. Just keep doing it. Try it for at least three minutes. See if any sounds come up that you have a desire to repeat, and if that happens, go with it. Otherwise, just keep experimenting with switching up the vowel sounds. Try not to form actual words that make sense to you — just raw sounds with no meaning. Feel the way they vibrate in the body.

This is not something you should try to make sense of with your mind. Thoughts do not matter. Instead, *feel* it. The sound energy you are sending into the universe is going to activate creation. You focus it on what feels harmonious and pleasurable in your body. The universe will show you the seeds that this energy germinates.

Chapter 7

Learning How to Read Your Body

Woman is the source of creation.

— DR. SARITA SHRESTHA, Ayurvedic ob-gyn from Nepal

In order for you and your partner to produce a healthy child, it's helpful if both of you are healthy, but we will initially discuss balancing *your* health, since you are of first importance. When your own body is aligned, then you can clearly see your partner, and you will be able to move forward together to consciously build your future life.

According to Ayurveda, the healthier you are, the more likely you are to be able to conceive a child, and also the healthier your child may be. There are mind-body enhancement practices, rasayanas, for both the mother and the father before conceiving a child together. Remember, health is not just about body, but mind and emotions, too. Balancing *yours* according to the principles you are learning in this book will help you achieve the best possible health prior to conception. Your partner must also align his own health. Then the two of you will produce excellent seed (ovum and sperm), which will be fit for the creative energy to enter.

Ayurveda's Indicators of Fertility

- Freedom from diseases, laziness, and greed
- Aliveness of senses
- Good-quality voice
- Strong libido

Following a wholesome diet and lifestyle, where you are in tune with your body type, life stage, environment, and seasons, is the key to preparing your body for conception. But before we go into specific practices for doing so, it's important to get you in the mental game first.

The Mental Game

By trying to develop more self-mastery, you will improve your health, and your overall life will get better. The yogis and yoginis throughout the centuries have passed down such great wisdom for developing self-mastery, guided by some pretty awesome philosophical texts and a mix of different characters who have dedicated their lives to teaching people this discipline. Practices such as mindfulness and various types of meditation are also modern ways that people try to get ahold of the animal they are riding around in — the body! Anything you do that helps you be more aware of your thoughts, feelings, and actions and shift any harmful or outdated patterns is beneficial to your mental game.

Making a decision to have a baby requires that you direct your focus toward the steps of this effort, and once you are there — you are in it! To prep your body well, you need to set your personal foundation first. The key is discipline, purification, and sensory-energy balancing. When your mind is clear, referred to as a *sattvic* state of being, you will trust yourself, concentrate your attention, make things happen, and then lose yourself in the experience.

But the mental game sometimes is challenging when there are imbalances and toxicity in a body. The mere presence of the imbalance prevents us from seeing clearly and colors our thoughts. If we balance the body, the mind becomes clearer. If the mind becomes clearer, it makes better choices that result in a more balanced body. This is known as *sattva*.

Reading the Tea Leaves of Your Cycle

Roughly every month, women are undergoing an all-out assault on their state of being by a little bit of biological programming that has been passed down from generation to generation. It's the cycle designed to make women the receptive hosts to a winning sperm that will forever change their lives. It's the cycle designed to make a lady sexy at just the right time, and then to flush the body of the supports it provided when that winning sperm doesn't show up or doesn't succeed in its mission. It's the cycle that drives a woman nuts from around age twelve to age fifty. Once you get it, you are generally stuck with it for a long time — well, that is, unless you start tinkering with various chemicals to stop it or your body becomes so depleted that it shuts it off naturally.

You can learn so much by observing what you are putting into your body, what it feels like inside there, and then what your body is putting out. It's worthwhile to study the whole body on a regular basis, like looking at your tongue and your waste products every day. It is also a good idea to study your moment-to-moment interactions — what's coming in contact with your senses, how you are interpreting information, and the actions you are putting back into your environment. In addition, once a month, you have an opportunity to receive the equivalent of a report card of your life experience. The menstrual cycle tells you much about how your life went during the time leading up to your monthly period. Whether your cycle feels smooth, blocked, intense, painful, heavy, light, or what have you — you will find out a great deal of what you need to know about your overall health in the functioning of your period. This alone makes your period worth all the challenges it brings.

Your overall body and your reproductive system have to be moderately healthy in order for you to have a baby. This does not mean you need to be perfect. "Perfect" doesn't exist, but the point is that it is better if you are healthy — for you and for a baby. A lot changes during and after pregnancy, so establishing a good foundation is important. Health means that your tissues are formed well, channels are flowing properly (not blocked, inflamed, malformed, or overactive), and the body can perform the functions it needs to in order to sustain your day-to-day lifestyle and potentially the life of a fetus.

Even if your reproductive tissues are fine, a major health issue in another region or system of the body can cause problems in your reproductive functioning as well, as discussed in chapter 5. You are a whole person, and all your organs are interdependent. That being said, let's make sure you have the best health possible so you can feel your best at all times.

Learning what the doshas look like in the phases of the menstrual cycle is like reading the tea leaves for your fertility. It will teach you more about your health, choices, and environment, because each cycle represents what happened to your body in the weeks and months prior.

Phase 1: Building (Water + Earth Elements)

The first phase of the cycle involves tissue growth. All growth in the body involves the earth element, and water contains the hormones that stimulate growth. This is when the batches of follicles housing eggs are growing after being in a resting state since the woman was inside her own mother's belly. These follicles are growing and competing to be the winning egg released in that cycle. Multiple eggs are growing out of their cozy homes in the ovary at the same time, but the first one to be released from it in this cycle is the one that stands a chance at getting fertilized (cases of more than one are rare).

This phase begins right after menstruation ends and is typically a time of calm energy for a woman's reproductive functioning, but underneath the surface, her body is building structures and preparing to make her seed available for contact with the world. This phase begins even before the last menstrual cycle, since the growth of the follicles is happening in waves and stages within the ovary and is not solely limited to the current cycle. Women who have vata and/or kapha imbalances sometimes get stuck in this stage. It's a cooler part of the cycle, and if a woman's body runs on the cold or slow-building side, then this may be a longer phase for her because it will take more time for her to heat up for the next phase of intensity and transformation.

Phase 2: Transformation (Fire + Water Elements)

The time around ovulation is known as the transformation phase. Growth manifests for each batch of follicles once ovulation is successful for one from the group. As with the building phase, water is present because it transports hormones, but fire increases in the transformation phase. The fire's heat releases the egg from the ovary, and it enters the fallopian tube. This is when the corpus luteum in the egg begins to produce and emit progesterone. This surge in progesterone causes the uterine lining to thicken in preparation for a potential pregnancy. The blood is a home site of pitta, and this excess of blood filling the uterus means pitta is naturally increasing.

After a few days of the egg hanging out in the fallopian tube and being shepherded toward the blood-filled uterus, there are two potential paths: The first is if a sperm penetrates the ovum and conception takes place. On this path, the blood that was filling the uterus will be used to begin building more tissues if implantation occurs. The second path is if the egg's corpus luteum simply dies off and stops producing progesterone, which initiates the next phase.

The transformation phase is the start of a more volatile period of the cycle. It is a time of intensity and heightened awareness — sometimes in many aspects of life, not just in the reproductive system. Passion is what makes a woman feel aroused and stimulates the attraction for her partner. Procreation is one of the main biological purposes of the menstrual cycle, and heat creates that passion for procreation.

The fire element first transforms the follicle surrounding the egg into the corpus luteum, which causes the egg to be released from its decades-long home in the ovary. Without fire, there can be no transformation — no release of the egg to meet its potential match and no heightened sensory awareness, such as smell, for her to scope or sniff out a potential mate. (What else would be the biological explanation for a woman's body temperature being raised during ovulation — to attract more mosquitoes?) Second, the uterus undergoes its own transformation in this stage, filling with blood — predominantly made up of the fire and water elements — to prepare for possible pregnancy.

Many women with imbalances due to a high fire element will find themselves with inflammatory issues beginning around the time following ovulation, and the inflammation may get more intense until the body releases blood during menstruation — the next phase of the cycle. Upticks in psoriasis or acne before the period are examples of this. Vascular issues will also become aggravated. This is the classic pitta-imbalanced woman. She may start experiencing flare-ups way before she gets her period and then feel a sense of relief during menstruation. For the unbalanced woman, PMS can seem to last forever!

If you know that the fire element naturally goes up midmonth, and you know how to balance this element, then you can build routines into your life that keep your pitta in check.

Phase 3: Destruction (Space + Air Elements)

When the menstrual cycle begins, any uterine lining that had built up to support a potential embryo in that current cycle is broken down, and its contents — blood and other fluids — are released from the uterus via the small hole in the cervix and then through the vagina into whatever feminine-hygiene product a woman chooses. Bleeding is usually a clear signal that a destruction phase is underway, though in the case of spotting or frequent bleeding, it could also be due to uterine-blood overflow from a high-pitta transformation phase. A woman may also be in a destruction phase and have little blood to show for it during menstruation, indicating that pitta is very low in the reproductive system.

The destruction phase is kicked off by a few events. The corpus luteum surrounding the egg starts to expire, and the body knows that the egg will be expiring soon, too. When the uterine lining is full, the lack of space causes a compression that incites a reaction — the uterus needs to clear out to create space again and may squeeze the blood out by contracting. The air element of vata is what causes waves of contracting, or cramping, and moves the blood and fluids of the lining, eroding them and causing them to excrete and flow through the cervix with gravity. Many women feel painful cramps, headaches, and digestive issues during this phase, and oftentimes this is because the body resists the flow of a stronger downward pull of gravity, which is necessary for blood to be released. It can also be due to the thickness of the lining, which is stubborn to move. When something restricts movement and flow, pain is a common symptom — pain due to backed-up pressure can occur even in other parts of the body. Ideally, the fire and water elements help liquefy the uterine lining so that menstruation moves fluidly.

Quick Reproductive Self-Evaluation

- If periods are very heavy, then look at pitta.
- If they are of short duration, low flow, or dry (brown or black), then look at vata.
- If they are very painful, look at vata and/or kapha.

It is important to note that ama — toxicity — can also be present in all these situations.

Much the way water evaporates from the earth to form clouds in the sky, only to rain back down to cool the earth, the menstrual cycle is a monthly water cycle that cleanses the woman's body and mind. Menstruation is like rain. There is a clear sky afterward, and the ground becomes fresh. The destruction allows for a reopening to possibility — something is lost, but in the release, space for new opportunity is gained.

Got a Troublesome Phase?

Most women tend to have more discomforts in the transformation and destructive phases, and the building phase is often more comfortable. Studying your body in each of the phases can inform you about the type of imbalances you are experiencing so you can adjust your diet and lifestyle accordingly.

EXERCISE: REPRODUCTIVE SELF-EVALUATION

Grab a notebook or journal, and write down answers to the following questions. Note anything unique about your period or reproductive functioning.

Timing/Duration of Menstrual Cycle

1. Number of days between the start of one period and the next?
2. Is the length of your cycle consistent or erratic?
3. How many days does your period usually last?
4. When was the first day of your last period?
5. When is the expected first day of your next period?
6. Do you consistently ovulate at the same time in your cycle each month?
7. What signs do you notice when you are ovulating?
8. Do you ever have spotting or bleeding between periods?

Blood Quality

9. What color is your menstrual blood?
10. Do you tend to have any clotting, membranes, mucus?
11. Does your blood stain your clothes or wash off fairly easily?

Blood Quantity

12. On your heaviest day, how many tampons/pads/cups do you use?

13. How many days do you bleed heavily?

Discomfort

14. Do you experience any cramping, headaches, water retention, bloating, irritability, or back pain during your cycle?

15. Do you experience any discomfort during or after sexual activity?

Sexual Activity

16. Are you sexually active? If so, how frequently, and at what time of day do you typically have sex?

17. Do you use birth-control pills, creams, patches, or an IUD or other device?

18. Do you apply any lubrication? If so, what kind?

19. Are you following any natural fertility-planning methods? If so, which ones?

20. Have you had sex during your period?

21. Are there certain times of the month when you feel more aroused?

Other

22. Anything else you've noticed about your cycles, fertility, or sex drive?

23. Do you notice specific smells during any phases of your cycle?

Your cycle teaches you about the state of your physical, mental, and emotional health, as influenced by your life and behaviors. If any one of these areas is suffering, the cycle will tell you. Once you have read the current cycle, you can take actions to position yourself optimally to care for your health, fertility, and overall life. This is useful not only for you but also for the baby you may be taking care of at some point.

Transformation is going to happen, whether you want it to or not. It's your job to allow it if you want to be fertile. This is how nature works, so understanding the typical shifts in your biology each month will help you deal with them with less pain and more grace.

Stopping Unhealthy Practices

As discussed in chapter 1, women are increasingly waiting to have kids until later so that they can do other things in their lives — build a career, make money, travel, and so forth — but most of these same women still want to have sex whenever they feel like it. They are able to achieve this thanks to pharmacological developments and medical technology. Birth-control measures range from pills, patches, rings or chips, condoms, IUDs, creams, and sponges to cycle tracking and the age-old withdrawal method. The research on whether any of these methods causes side effects is quite all over the place, but Ayurveda tells us that we have to keep channels open in order for energy to flow.

Implanting drugs that block cellular transport at a micro level, or physical objects to block the passage of sperm and liquids, always carries the risk of interfering with biological functions or causing irritation — especially in areas designed to have fluids flow through them very regularly. On top of this, chemically or physically altering the blood or fluids of the body to trigger hormone changes — regardless of whether the route of application is oral or through the skin — has not only a local but also a systemic effect. Anytime we interfere with a normal, natural biological process in trying to meet a narrowly focused goal, there is always a danger of it causing some sort of imbalance more broadly in the body, because we've lost sight of the bigger picture. This is one of the basic principles behind *holistic* therapies, which help us see how things are interconnected by considering the mental, physical, emotional, behavioral, and environmental factors that influence imbalance and disease.

Birth-control methods can cause disrupted, irritated, or blocked reproductive tissues. For example, physically implanting or placing objects inside the body (such as chips, rings, or hormonal IUDs) for extended periods of time can cause irritation and block fluids from freely flowing where they need to go naturally. Also, chemically interfering with the natural processes of the menstrual cycle (via pills, patches, rings, chips, or hormonal IUDs) carries the risk of unintentionally altering other parts of the body and causing systemic changes, which then will affect the reproductive tissues.

A woman's sexual practices can also be disruptive to her reproductive tissue and result in problems with her menstrual cycles. For example, having sex without proper lubrication of the vagina (using lubricated condoms, creams, lubes) can cause inflammation and tissue damage. This can be due to lack of arousal, having sex too late in the cycle, dosha imbalance, or other toxicity. In addition, blocking or reversing excretion, such as when a woman has sex while menstruating or holds bowel movements, can cause a pressure backup (reversal of the apana vayu, or downward wind current), potentially displacing blood flow or disrupting its direction or levels.

Part of the wisdom of being a woman is to know when it is biologically time for sex and when it is not. Having sex when the body is focusing on other tasks is an example of kala parinama, or not being in harmony with nature's cycles, which was described earlier as one of the three main causes of disease. Nevertheless, many women do this because either their calendars or their mental-emotional desires and cravings have been driving their lives instead of the body's natural wisdom.

You can make a mistake here and there. The less time that goes by during which you allow a crime against nature to be committed, the easier it is to get back into balance. The body is forgiving. However, if any of these behaviors are causing health issues, and you continue them for an extended period, then you may be causing long-term damage to your body. Ayurveda provides another level of relief for those of us who have gotten out of balance — we can oftentimes heal from such issues with proper detoxification if we have not allowed it to go too far.

Many women today are waiting until they want to have a child before getting off their birth control. Other women can tell that something about it does not feel right, or they may have read about the side effects. At some point, all these women will stop their birth-control method, and they may want to take steps to move to a natural fertility-planning method while detoxing their bodies.

Natural Fertility Planning

A woman can study her cycles to either promote or prevent pregnancy. There are different fertility-planning techniques popular today that you may have already come across, such as the rhythm method, fertility awareness methods, and the Creighton Model, in which women try to predict the stage of their cycle based on either timing or physiological cues. The common theme in all these methods is that you are trying to understand where your body is in its cycle and align your actions based on your intentions, though in each method, the data points you are using to determine fertility are slightly different.

1. You can count the number of days from your first period and estimate when you think you are ovulating — if you have a sense of your normal ovulation patterns.

2. You can check your cervical mucus to note if the consistency of vaginal fluid has become runnier, more slippery and/or stretchy (a sign of ovulation) or has dried up (signaling a less fertile phase).

3. You can put your finger way up inside your vagina and see if the position of the cervix has changed — if dropped, then more fertile; and if high, then less fertile.

4. You can track your body temperature and see when it spikes during ovulation, as research shows that both body

temperature and level of physical activity increase in some species at ovulation.

All these methods allow you to get to know your body, because all these changes are typical of ovulation. However, there are some potential challenges with each of these methods.

First, a woman who has high kapha may be juicy all the time and may not even notice much of a change in her vaginal fluid. A woman who has high vata may not notice ovulation because she is always on the drier side, and a woman with high pitta may not notice any difference in her body temperature if she's constantly feeling hot. Counting the days from the start of her last period does a woman no good if her biological markers of ovulation are confusing and she has no clue when she typically ovulates. The body doesn't follow a calendar the way the mind wants it to, but if you get to know *your* normal and *your* unique signs, then you are more likely to know where you are in your cycle.

Now here's the challenge: though there are general patterns to all female menstrual cycles, a fair amount of variation can occur from month to month. Regularity depends on birth constitution, life stage, and seasonal and lifestyle factors, such as diet and sleep. Major life transitions will affect your cycles. Even your relationship and work stability will affect them. Understanding the functioning and influencers of your biology can help you establish a lifestyle and sexual practices that align with your intentions to either prevent or enable conception. Learn your patterns, and pay attention to changes.

How the Reproductive System Gets Nourishment

The reproductive materials of the body are the last to get nourishment. The parts of the body needed for basic life functions demand nourishment first, and if there is anything left over when all those priority functions are covered, then the body sends nourishment to the reproductive material. In addition, the quality and frequency of the nourishment will either enable healthy reproductive functioning or impede it. Too much nourishment, wrong nourishment, or nourishment at the wrong times can clog and block channels, cause inflammation, and hinder the receptivity of the body. Therefore, proper nourishment of the woman's body is needed to support a potential new life.

Sex can be a depleting act in a body that is already depleted. If you find yourself in this category, it's important to make sure that your diet replenishes the fluids and nutrients lost. Drinking room-temperature or warm water and eating foods like ghee, dates, and almonds can help replenish a depleted reproductive system. Fennel seeds, aloe, and cinnamon will bring more fluids and energy to the reproductive area.

If your body is improperly nourished or carrying cloudy, heavy, dense energy, this can slow or block the transport of blood and fluids, as well as cellular communication, possibly even causing growths in reproductive tissues. What you eat becomes your tissues. And since like increases like, you want to take in the qualities that you need to be healthy. You can essentially design how your reproductive system gets nourished.

The timing of when you eat in relation to sex matters. The blood and fluids that go to the reproductive system during sex will be infused with whatever quality is already circulating in the blood. Similarly, the blood and fluids that fill the uterus right after ovulation will have been influenced by what you ate and drank around that time. It's better to keep your body balanced and healthy so that the nourishment is of good quality when it travels to the reproductive system. In general, it's preferable to eat after sex, rather than before, so that the digestive system isn't working so hard while you are trying to get energy in your reproductive organs. However, you might take an herbal medicine before sex if your intent were to deliver the herb to the reproductive area.

Furthermore, if you follow a diet and lifestyle appropriate to your particular constitutional type and life demands (covered more in the following chapter), then you are more likely to have equilibrium in your reproductive functioning. If your environment is free from toxicity, even better. This is health. And if you have a partner whom you feel ready to have a child with, you may consider yourself to be in good shape to prepare for conception.

Deep-Dive Practices

Denying yourself something that you typically derive pleasure from can increase your appreciation of it. It can also help you notice more of your body's signals, because there are fewer external influences to factor in.

Sex Fast

If you and your partner are used to having regular sex, then it may be helpful to take a pause together and experiment with a sex fast. The way you go about it is to refrain from having sex for a month, the entire duration of one of your menstrual cycles, or a different time frame of your choosing. The reason you are doing this is to start to read the body and observe some of the following:

- *When do I get aroused — are there certain times of day or certain times of the month? What triggers arousal for me?*
- *What are some body sensations I feel when I am aroused?*
- *How frustrated do I get when I cannot have sex when I want to?*
- *Do I want to have sex more or less frequently than I thought?*
- *Where do I put my energy when I'm not having sex?*

Simply taking this time off will give you and your partner a lot of really cool information. However, you both have to be on board with this idea, and neither should take any of the findings personally. Libido is very much influenced by diet, lifestyle, and individual history, and at the same time, with a little attention and inspiration, it can be consciously cultivated.

A sex fast can have other benefits. One example is that men who ejaculate less frequently can actually improve the number of viable sperm, and this can be important because men's sperm counts have collectively decreased significantly in the last half century. Therefore, when the sex fast is broken, your partner may have increased potency — so hold on to your hat!

Fasting from sex can give you an opportunity to see what happens to your cycles when your body is mainly dealing with its own physical energy. There is typically also a pleasurable side effect: adding a very small amount of space between you and your partner can oftentimes increase the level of sensitivity experienced. On the other hand, remember that you must have sex to have a baby, so don't practice a sex fast for too long if you want to conceive!

Fasting from Food

If you are not sure if you need to balance out your body more, or if you are uncertain about moving forward with motherhood, then it's time to take a deeper dive: fasting from food. I imagine it may sound somewhat contradictory to fast when you are thinking about getting pregnant, but for many women, fasting while preparing for conception is a common, very powerful practice. When you are creating something, matter is shifting. The easiest way to shift matter in your body is to experiment with different eating rituals. But before we go forward, I have to stop right here to clarify that there are some instances in which you should not explore fasting.

It's not a great idea to fast if you are underweight or undernourished or if you have certain medical conditions. I'm providing this option assuming that many of the women who read this book are robust enough to be able to tolerate and even benefit from a little fasting here and there. Fasting is not appropriate for individuals with eating disorders. It is not recommended for women who are breastfeeding or who have become pregnant. It's also best to skip fasting on the days when you are ovulating, because it will intensify that time frame without providing the adequate nourishment to counterbalance the intensity. You may consult with your doctor or healthcare practitioner prior to exploring fasting if you are concerned about any of these points.

If you are still here, let's proceed. The Sanskrit word used to refer to fasting from something is *upavāsa*, which means, more literally, "to stay close to one's soul." Fasting is one way for you to begin diving deeper into that primal space inside, where all creative energy resides.

The ancient Ayurvedic medical text *Charaka-samhita*, which was written around 600 BCE, indicates that fasting is a preparatory measure an individual should take when about to study with a master. This is because fasting creates a more receptive body, mind, and spirit. The master you are about to study with, in this case, is Mother Nature. You will begin to see her as ever more present in your own body, in the world around you, and in the processes that bring a child into the world.

I find that most of my clients are eating three meals a day and snacks between meals, but oftentimes it is not an eating pattern that would work best for an individual's body with today's lifestyles. Frequently, this eating pattern can actually decrease the metabolic capability and clog various vital channels of the body with toxins, while simultaneously taxing the digestive system and stealing energy from other areas that need it. Once a body becomes toxic, flow is interrupted and bodily imbalances like degeneration, inflammation, or pathological growth conditions occur, as we touched on earlier.

Why are people eating like this when it's actually causing illness in so many? A lot of people were misled at some point, told that this is what they are "supposed" to do. Others used to feel more hunger at a different stage of their lives and simply haven't shifted to meet the current demands. Others are working so hard that their hunger is insatiable and they simply need more rest. In addition, most people are not comfortable feeling a little hungry when they have such easy and affordable access to food. In some cases people are mistaking appetite and craving for hunger, so they believe they need the food, but they are misreading the body's signals.

Mentally, when a woman never experiences true biological hunger, she does not know what her response to it will be. If you are used to eating regularly, then you may not have felt true hunger for a while. People who fast often characterize the mental struggle as being worse than any physical struggle they feel. While there can be some discomfort in fasting, most individuals in a developed society today have enough stored fat and sugar in their bodies, which can get released into the bloodstream for use if they go into fat-burning mode due to fasting periods. In other words, most people's bodies have a big enough savings account to tap into when new food isn't coming in. In fact, one of the main benefits of fat-burning mode is the energy release from stored glycogen (glucose) and fatty acids (ketones) that is used to power the body. The ketones, especially, are described by many as an energy source that feels even more enlivening than glucose. This is one reason why individuals on a spiritual quest will fast. It appears that people like the buzz they get from it.

In addition, fasting redirects resources away from digestion toward other bodily functions that are essential, including the immune response to toxins and pathogens. So, oftentimes, if you eat a little less, your body can spend more time building up its resistance to harmful things it may come in contact with and clearing out blockages and poorly formed tissues. On the other hand, if you fast too much, the side effects — including compromised agni, tissue depletion, and even inflammation — can be detrimental to your overall and reproductive health. In preparing for conception, you want to be an open channel, but not an inflamed open channel.

Fasting increases wavelike motions in the body and, when done well, can also heighten one's intensity and agni. Some people notice that if they eat a little less frequently, it actually increases the number of bowel movements they have. This happens because when we first start to eat less, the body goes into a primal cleansing and clearing mode so that we can be light on our feet and find the next food source.

You are, after all, trying to tap into that primal, animal place inside — so if you end up turning into a more dramatic version of yourself, this is not necessarily a bad thing. This is your animal self; it wants to survive. A well-fed body oftentimes becomes very comfortable, but it also runs the risk of becoming stagnant and stuck. (I can still hear the voice of one of my teachers in Ayurveda school in my head, telling the class over and over again how creation comes from turbulence.) On the other hand, if fasting is practiced too much, it can end up reducing agni and ruining your metabolic power so badly that you might need to take special herbs just to rekindle the agni. Finding the balance is key.

EXERCISE: THE FASTING EXPERIMENT

The purpose of this experiment is to explore and test your boundaries and invoke the energies of creation — creating a little space invites new matter. It isn't meant to be anything extreme, though it *is* intended to raise your awareness, and some individuals typically suffering from really growly, burning stomachs or missed periods, and those who are underweight or have a serious medical condition should skip this experiment.

Wake up in the morning at your usual time and do not eat until you get ravenously hungry, to the point where you feel your stomach burn or growl a little. See how long you can go without having a bunch of physical discomfort, and then eat the meal that you normally would during that part of the day. Some people will find that they are hungry very early in the day, and this means that their agni is strong. Others will find they don't actually get hungry until lunchtime, and this means that the agni is weak, or slow. Your agni can be too weak or too sharp, and the object is to find what is balanced agni for your body.

If you practice fasting for a while, you may notice that new cravings appear. Listen to these. A craving that comes up because you are used to it is much different from one that comes up out of nowhere. The former is habitual, and the latter is a true craving. For example, I've had cravings for chocolate while fasting because I was used to eating chocolate all the time, and then I've had cravings for random foods that I hadn't eaten for years, like eggplant parmigiana, which was a dish I was never really crazy about. Suddenly I just had to have eggplant parmigiana. Fasting helps you dive deep into your body, where both your cellular memory and your psyche may bring up some odd things that surprise you. Try to understand what is behind the craving, and satisfy it. Your body has wisdom it's sharing with you.

The Importance of Reading Your Body

As we've already learned, health is a state of balanced biological humors, properly formed tissues, moderate hunger, and a clear mind and senses. Paying attention to your body's excretions — stool, urine, sweat, blood, tears, vaginal fluid, and so on — is important. You may notice odd qualities sometimes, such as a different quantity of excreta, dryness, burning, a smell, or even blood where it shouldn't normally be. These are all symptoms of imbalance in your body. Your skin will sometimes show you that something is wrong as well — dryness, acne, red rashes, swelling, or dandruff — and possibly indicative of a more systemic issue. You want healthy tissues and flowing channels, so adopting lifestyle behaviors that align you with your best health is key.

Similarly, in your fertility, it is important to read your body's cues. Desire and arousal are essential for healthy sexual intercourse. Don't have sex just to get pregnant. If you aren't feeling physical desire, yet your mind is saying you want to have a baby, then there is a clear disconnect between mind and body that you must address. When you're trying to make a baby naturally, your body's urges trump your mind's. What happens if you have sex when you aren't aroused? It hurts, doesn't it? Adding lubricants is simply masking the fact that, while your mind may want to have sex, your body does not. If you have sex at that time, then you are actually risking injuring your tissues. If you want to get pregnant naturally, it's worth it for your body to be on board with the plan!

If any of this is speaking to you even a little, it's critical for you to do some further soul-searching on your state of balance: your work-life balance, relationship with your partner, and overall mind-body health. Remember, the body is *intelligent*.

The ability to read the body becomes very important later, once a baby is born, because a baby cannot talk to tell you something is wrong. You must read the baby's body, smells, sounds, and so on. Therefore, learning how to read your own body is a very handy skill for a mom-to-be!

If you are still feeling confused about your own health, don't worry. In the following chapter, you'll learn even more about the doshas and how they can be balanced with Ayurveda.

Chapter 8

Healing Fertility Rituals and Practices

Our bodies are ideally designed and adapted to carry,
give birth to and nourish our young just like any other mammal,
and yet, unlike other mammals, we appear to be the only species
which has difficulty in fulfilling our instinctive potential.

— **JANET BALASKAS**, *Preparing for Birth with Yoga*

Life experiences plant a type of seed inside your memory. These experiences are collected, their impressions recorded and stored away for future use. The Sanskrit term *samskara* is an imprint left on the mind. Your whole life you are collecting these imprints, though it's not something that you do consciously. Imprints are simply the result of a life lived, of being in the world, having experiences, seeing things, and so forth. The imprints are placed inside you and stored as a seed in your memory waiting for future activation. These seeds can go unnoticed for a long time if your life conditions lack the triggers that normally activate them and bring them back to your awareness. If the tides turn, and the environment presents a trigger, the seed may become activated.

This same mechanism that happens in the mind also happens in the body. The body becomes programmed. It has memory. It remembers pleasure and it remembers pain. It also gets physically wounded sometimes. When a tissue becomes wounded — due to either injury or a behavioral cause — it is said to create a *khavaigunya*, or an injured, weak, or defective space in the body. When the doshas get out of balance and start traveling through a body, it's in these weak spots that they find the opportunity to slip in and create imbalance. Healthy tissues, on the other hand, are better able to protect themselves. Sometimes trouble spots are created before birth and other times afterward, but either way, they can be exacerbated when the body gets out of balance in the future. We all have them, and they are to be treated with care.

What this means is that if you have an imbalance process in place prior to trying to conceive, it's possible that it will be affected when your body is inevitably thrown out of whack from pregnancy. It could go either way — the imbalance could get better or worse. On the other hand, because trouble spots and imbalances can also prevent further normal functioning if they interfere with vital channels — blood and lymphatic vessels, nerves, cellular transport, and so on — they sometimes need to be cleansed, healed, and rejuvenated prior to any attempt to conceive.

If you have imbalances, weak spots, or wounds, then it is important to get to know them before you have a child. If you decide to try to heal any imbalances beforehand, please do so with sensitivity and patience. Getting care from a professional and developing a supportive network around you in these cases is essential. With proper care, problem areas can sometimes be healed and rejuvenated, and if that is not possible, then they can at least be managed, which is much better than having them continue to get worse.

I've known many people who instinctively could tell there was something off with their bodies, but because they had no name for it, they didn't believe themselves. Sometimes even their doctors brushed off their complaints because they weren't presenting as clearly manifested diseases. However, it's beneficial to pay attention early when there are imbalances, and I'm hoping this book gives you some terms and concepts to represent sensations you may not have had words to describe well in the past, like I found happening to me when I started studying Ayurveda.

Practices for Your Dominant Dosha(s)

You are an individual, so first let me say that it would be a mistake to assume that you are simply a body type, as we aspiring Ayurvedis often do. On the other hand, there are patterns that appear in people's bodies and minds with the doshas, and balancing these patterns can be very helpful in preparing for conception. In addition to taking into account the doshas, we have to consider your life stage and your environmental conditions, including the season of the year. This chapter contains rasayanas, which are mind-and-body-enhancing therapies for each dosha type during the preconception period.

This time before conception is a pause to get your proverbial ducks in a row. It's important to do this before, rather than while, you are pregnant, because *how* something is initially created has a tremendous effect on its overall life trajectory. In addition, it's sometimes not safe to do certain body-balancing practices if you are already pregnant, and if you experience an imbalance, you may end up getting stuck with it until after you give birth or in some cases until after breastfeeding ends. A woman's body goes through mind-blowing changes, so starting off on the healthiest footing is always best.

Remember that your life stage, the time of year, and even the general climate you live in may naturally drive up one or more of the doshas. You can't change the weather, but you can learn to adapt your practices and lifestyle to it. You can't reverse or speed up time, but you can be the healthiest version of yourself in each life stage. It's up to you to adapt appropriately.

If you know something is off in your body, then I recommend that you spend at least ninety days on rebalancing. If you can dedicate six months, all the better. If there are stronger or longer-term imbalances, it may take more time and additional care, cleansing, and rejuvenation for the changes to stick. By the end of this chapter, I hope you will have selected a couple of the rituals and practices that you think will help you balance your mind-body-spirit, based on what you've learned in this book and through other insights you've had in your life — and I recommend that you commit to these practices and rituals for at least a few months before you try to conceive. Your body doesn't change as quickly as your mind does, so it needs more time to adjust.

Let's begin.

Recognizing and Addressing Vata Dominance

If you've been experiencing any of the cardinal signs of a vata imbalance listed below, you can follow the vata-dominant preconception practices. These practices involve revitalization and restoring groundedness, strength, stability, warmth, and juiciness to the body.

General Signs of a Vata Imbalance

- Anxiety, fear, memory issues, or general feeling of being scattered and unfocused
- Insomnia
- Constipation
- Dry asthma
- Eczema
- Joint pain
- Dry skin
- Muscle spasms, irregular heartbeats, or twitching feelings
- Roughness or lack of juiciness
- Dehydration

We need vata. It's the source of movement, which is good for creation. However, since too much vata is a "breaking down" state, it is the opposite of the kind of state you will be in if you become pregnant. This is a tricky balance, though, because you also do not want to correct your vata so radically that you start to increase pitta and kapha too much. Therefore, with vata, the best strategies are to slow down, rest, and create rejuvenating routines.

If you recall, earlier in the book we discussed how the qualities of vata include *cold, dry, light, rough, subtle, mobile,* and *clear.* Does it seem like you have too much of any of these qualities? One simple tweak to your daily routines is to fill your environment and your diet with foods, sounds, smells, and materials that oppose the quality that is out of balance. For example, if you're experiencing dryness and roughness, then you likely need more slimy and oily textures. If you're eating a diet full of dry popcorn, crackers, and beans, then this will dry you out and crack the tissues. Eat some oily, salty soups and some sautéed veggies to nourish the depleted, dehydrated tissues and plump them up. More vata qualities in your diet will increase vata in your body. Reducing vata qualities in your diet reduces vata in your body.

Energy needs to go to the reproductive area for optimal functioning. Too much vata causes rapid aging and degeneration and can result in dry, scanty periods, irregular cycles, and early menopause, while too little vata will slow the system down and block overall functioning of the menstrual cycles.

SIGNS OF A HIGH-VATA REPRODUCTIVE SYSTEM

- Very early or very late menarche (first period)
- Irregular cycles (no clear pattern or abnormal cycle)
- Absent periods (amenorrhea)
- Very light periods or brown-colored periods (indicating dryness)
- Brief body-temperature spikes during ovulation
- Endometriosis (due to dispersing of endometrial tissue)
- Early menopause
- Lack of vaginal fluid upon arousal
- Gas, bloating, and low-back spasms before onset of menstruation
- Feelings of fear, anxiety, and worry; mood swings; or mania during menstruation
- Disinterest in sex (due to depletion)

Quick, mobile, erratic lifestyles, along with eating or coming in contact with too many cold, hard, dry, rough, or light foods or environmental qualities, will raise vata. A woman who lacks commitment and has difficulty forming lasting intimate relationships with people will oftentimes have high vata, since there is an increase of space and a decrease of grounding and attachment.

Women who travel a lot for work or other reasons can experience disruption in their cycles because of the overall increased movement and also because flying and driving can both raise vata and aggravate existing imbalances. In addition, as stated earlier, major life alterations, such as a relationship change, a new job, or moving residences, will raise vata. Women in these transition states often experience disruptions in their menstrual cycle. We are unfathomably deeply connected to the environment and people around us.

In my practice, whenever a woman comes to me with an irregular menstrual cycle, my first line of questioning is often about lifestyle and routines, and inevitably I will hear a story about a recent divorce, breakup, job change, or trip somewhere. The good thing is that once the person's life stabilizes, and routines are reestablished, the irregularity typically quiets down or even disappears within only a month or two.

The following section includes rasayanas for vata: dietary and lifestyle recommendations for a woman with a vata imbalance, plus recommendations for mind-body practices, body treatments, and helpful herbs. A woman can dabble in some of them or try all of them, but the key is to implement these changes and follow them with as much consistency as possible until vata is balanced.

Vata-Balancing Dietary and Lifestyle Practices

BALANCING QUALITIES TO EXPLORE

Warm, oily, heavy, dull, gross, static, and cloudy

DIET

Eat regularly, at least every 3–4 hours. The size of the meal depends on the degree of hunger, but keep a regular eating routine and have the largest meal around lunchtime. Try drinking ginger tea if not hungry at mealtimes in order to strengthen agni.

Favor:
- Cooked, moist foods, such as soups, stews, and well-cooked stir-fries
- Moderate to high amounts of oils and good fats (plant or animal based)
- Sweet, salty, and sour tastes
- Nourishing and sustaining foods
- Prunes and soaked raisins or almonds added to meals or snacks

Avoid:
- Raw vegetables
- Cold and iced foods and substances
- Drying foods and substances (like popcorn, beans, coffee, and alcohol)
- Extreme bingeing or starving behaviors

HERBS/SPICES

Some basic kitchen spices are very helpful for balancing vata. A little of the following spices/seasonings added to meals can help, especially if they are accompanied by some good oils. As a supplement, a pinch of these spices can be taken in a cup of warm water with one teaspoon of oil:

- Cinnamon
- Nutmeg
- Ginger
- Turmeric
- Salt

If these sound a bit like fall spices you might find in a pumpkin pie, that's because they are. Fall is vata season.

Herbal medicines can also be explored for stronger vata imbalances, but it's probably better to work with an Ayurvedic professional if dabbling in these because they can have stronger effects than many kitchen herbs, which means they can also have stronger side effects if used incorrectly:

- Shatavari + ashwagandha (together in equal parts)
- Haritaki
- Licorice (short-term use only)
- Dashamula (Ayurvedic formula of ten root herbs)
- Brahmi bacopa (*Bacopa monnieri*)
- Cedar
- Chyawanprash (herbal jam)

SLEEP

Develop a regular sleep routine with a set bedtime every night, preferably before 11, and if you can get to bed by 10, even better. Though vata-dominant people tend to feel that they need less sleep to function, not getting enough perpetuates the vata imbalance and can cause both bodily and mental dysfunction and degeneration.

If you need naps during the day, take them at the same time daily, but eventually get more sleep at night so you no longer need to nap during the day.

EXERCISE

First, it is important for vata-dominant people to make sure they do not exercise excessively, because although they may like to move, they will end up hurting themselves and becoming depleted. Instead, practice slow, warming, stabilizing types of exercise. Try slow yoga with long-held poses, Pilates, and resistance-based exercise, like lifting weights. Try to get warm and sweat a little but not excessively. Since vata is already dry, excessive sweat can make this worse. Even 10–15 minutes of exercise is sufficient, so do a little bit every day and prioritize rest more.

MIND-BODY PRACTICES

Vata-dominant people have difficulty with solo meditation practices and also need to be careful with some of the breathing practices done in yoga, because breathing a lot creates more dryness and movement in the body. Breath energy, *prana*, is vata, and you can actually have too much of it. Vata people are better served by focusing on their bodies, rather than their minds, and sitting and planning out their day, rather than practicing some sort of meditation on their own. Guided meditations, *yoga nidra,* and restorative yoga are very rejuvenating. Repeating affirmations or mantras silently is also helpful to balance vata.

BODY TREATMENTS

Oil massage on the body is often one of the first practices for vata-dominant people. The oil penetrates the skin and gets into the blood-stream and lymphatic channels. This lubricates, calms, and grounds the body. This can be done at home, as frequently as every day during very dry seasons, and perhaps only once or twice a week in less extreme conditions.

To do an oil massage, or *abhyanga,* at home, apply food-grade cooking oil, such as untoasted sesame or sunflower oil, to the skin all over the body, face, and scalp. Warm the oil slightly first so it does not feel cool when applied. Let the oil sit for anywhere from 5 to 30 minutes, and then take a nice warm shower to allow the oil to penetrate a little deeper while you gently wipe any excess oil off the skin. Abhyanga can be done either in the morning as a protective practice or before bed to promote restful sleep.

SEXUAL PRACTICES

Vata individuals can be on the dry side, so they must be adequately aroused for intercourse. Using lubricants can actually interfere with conception, so they are a last resort. It is better to rebalance your whole system and then have the reproductive tissue become naturally juicy. Vata people should conserve their energy and moisture, so they might find it more balancing for their bodies to have sex less frequently, maybe only a couple of times a month.

Vata-Balancing Daily Routine

Consistency is important, because vata-dominant people tend to lack solid routines. Practicing something at the same time every day, for example, equals consistency. Trying a change one day and then maybe again the following week is not consistent. Vata-dominant people need their daily schedules more structured. The body can relax more when there is more predictability. Vata-imbalanced people are probably more likely to take risks in life, but they have to watch that they don't do this too much, because they are also not usually the sturdiest of body types, which makes tolerating risk difficult.

So, for a vata-dominant individual, a sample daily routine might look like the following.

VATA-BALANCING DAILY SCHEDULE

TIME	ACTIVITY
7:00 AM	Waking up
7:15 AM	Drinking a cup of warm water, cinnamon, turmeric, sesame oil, and salt Hot shower
7:30 AM	Planning for the day and/or guided meditation
8:00 AM	Breakfast
11:00 AM	Lunch
3:00 PM	Snack
5:00 PM	Slow movement (tai chi, yoga) or weight-bearing exercise
7:00 PM	Dinner
9:30 PM	Application of warm-oil abhyanga Shower or bath
11:00 PM	Bedtime

This is just a rough example. If you are dealing with a vata imbalance, factor in your existing daily routines and sketch out a new, ideal hour-by-hour timeline that will help slow things down and rejuvenate you. Make sure to note regular work and recreational activities, including going out with friends, as I've found that many vata individuals seem to have difficulty establishing routines because they love being out on the town and aren't the best sleepers.

How doable does this feel to you? Vatas are best served by structure and reducing empty space and movement, so planning your day is one of the most beneficial things you can do.

The Role of Vata in Imbalance

It is said that an imbalance of vata is often at the root of pitta and kapha imbalances, because vata is behind all changes. Vata is made of space and air elements. Space, known as *akasha*, is essentially a vacuum or opportunity. Air, known as *vayu*, is an unseen force that drives the movement of matter. You can't see air, but you can see what it moves. You can see the humors of pitta (bile, bilirubin, and red blood, for example) and kapha (such as mucus or synovial fluid), but you can't see vata. You can see only its aftereffects.

You can hear vata moving through the digestive tract. The aftereffect of vata in a tissue is roughness, dryness, coldness, erosion, and the like, which then end up causing matter to stick to it more easily — while the aftereffect of pitta is heat, inflammation, spreading, sharpness, or redness, and the aftereffect of kapha is dampness, heaviness, slowness, and growths. The idea is that if a change or movement didn't occur in the first place, then neither pitta nor kapha would go out of balance. Oftentimes, when vata increases in the environment, a person may react or compensate for the extra movement and energy by taking in too many pitta or kapha qualities through the diet and senses. Other times pitta and kapha go out of balance because a person has failed to see their associated qualities start to increase in the environment.

Temperamentally, excess vata may elicit a fearful or anxiety-filled personality, but if a pitta increase follows, then a critical, problem-solving, action-oriented mentality will ensue. If kapha follows the vata increase, then so does the grasping mechanism in many people. Excess kapha is sticky, greedy, and clingy. However, without the extra movement and change of vata, pitta and kapha are less likely to go out of balance due to diet and lifestyle.

You can have too much vata if you are following a vata-exacerbating lifestyle or diet, and this is more likely to become further exacerbated in very cold or dry weather. This weather makes you more permeable and sucks the moisture and matter out of you. In addition, you can have too much vata if you have toxic blockages in your body. When channels become blocked, energy gets redirected to weird places where you will be able to feel it.

Recognizing and Addressing Pitta Dominance

When a woman has been overwhelmed by a pitta imbalance, she may feel anger and intensity and have signs of inflammation, such as redness, rashes, or acne; a sour-smelling body; super-heavy or frequent periods; heartburn; or even yellowish stool. Pitta-imbalanced individuals can also have difficulty falling asleep, because they are busy bees, but they oftentimes tire themselves out so that sleep is easier.

GENERAL SIGNS OF A PITTA IMBALANCE

- Anger, irritability, or general feelings of being too hot or intense
- Hot or burning upper or lower GI tract or urinary tract
- Loose and/or yellow stools
- Jaundice (yellowish color in the skin and/or eyes)
- Red acne or rashes
- Allergies
- Psoriasis
- Super-heavy or frequent periods
- Foul or sour body odor

If you've been experiencing signs of pitta imbalance, you can follow the pitta-dominant preconception practices. Inflammation can cause cells to become overreactive and can also reduce space in different channels of the body, so it can impede fertility. The body must be

receptive in order to conceive and gestate. These pitta-reducing practices involve cooling the body, expelling toxicity, creating space, and
slowing down. As stated earlier, a pitta state is a transformation state,
and transformation is the purpose of some of the processes enabled if
you become pregnant (the others are building processes and then later
releasing and supporting processes). Therefore, pitta imbalances will
often get worse during pregnancy as the blood volume increases, so it's
important to address them before conception.

The qualities of pitta include *hot, oily, light, sharp, mobile,* and *liquid.* Are any of these qualities feeling all too common for you? To balance pitta, you must choose to incorporate opposite qualities — in
your nutrition and what you take in through the five senses.

Pitta increases from intensity, heat, quickness, and sharp energy. A
woman's pitta rises naturally when she is ovulating and gets a release
valve each month with the menstrual cycle. It also increases when she
is pregnant, because it's pitta that is responsible for transmuting nutrients into tissues, both in the woman's body and in a growing baby
inside her. We need a certain level of heat in order to achieve ovulation
in the cycle, but too much heat can cause inflammation, very heavy or
frequent periods (including spotting), or damage to the tissues of the
reproductive tract.

Many women with inflammatory conditions, such as red, rashy skin
conditions, will find relief when menstruation finally starts, because
the release of uterine blood naturally reduces their overall blood volume, and thus their reproductive and systemic pitta also diminishes.
However, if the pitta imbalance is not resolved, then it will go right
back up above healthy levels at the ovulation peak in the next month.

It can feel very intense for a woman with high pitta in her reproductive tract. She may feel an insatiable physical desire for, or even irritability toward, sex throughout her cycle or be very annoyed by the amount
of blood she loses each month. The emotions of anger and resentment
and irritability are all associated with high pitta, and she radiates intensity into her environment, regardless of whether she expresses herself.
The best medicine for high pitta is slow, cooling downtime, which is
typically what a woman begins to crave during menstruation. If she

continues burning the midnight oil, so to speak, during this time, she may not find the relief her body and psyche both need.

Balancing pitta is important during the middle years of a woman's life, especially the transitions into and out of her fertile season. As a young woman moves from childhood to adulthood and puberty starts, you can frequently see the signs of increasing pitta. Menarche often occurs around the same time acne starts for some women. Children are naturally watery, but an adolescent begins to develop more fire, too. This is because the middle of life involves reproductive power and higher-pitta years. Women with excess pitta in their systems oftentimes experience an intense surge of bleeding during perimenopause, and it can be extra challenging for them at that time.

SIGNS OF A HIGH-PITTA REPRODUCTIVE SYSTEM IMBALANCE

- Early menarche
- More frequent cycles, spotting, or very heavy periods (menorrhagia)
- Body-temperature spikes during ovulation that remain higher for a longer period of time
- Inflammation of the vagina, the cervix, or other reproductive tissues
- Headache, acne breakout, or uptick in red skin conditions before onset of menstruation
- Feelings of intensity, anger, or resentment during premenstrual period
- Overwhelming interest in sex

The following section includes dietary and lifestyle recommendations for a woman with a pitta imbalance, plus recommendations for mind-body practices, body treatments, and helpful herbs.

Pitta-Balancing Dietary and Lifestyle Practices

BALANCING QUALITIES TO EXPLORE
Cold, dry, heavy, dull, static, and dense

Diet

Eat regularly, at least every 4–5 hours. The size of the meal depends on the degree of hunger, but keep a regular eating routine, because pitta individuals tend to have the strongest appetites, as they are burning through a lot of energy due to their dynamic, hot nature. It is important to eat when hungry because the secretions associated with hunger if it is not satisfied in a pitta body will damage the lining of the digestive tract.

Favor:
- A variety of cooling foods, including both raw and cooked foods
- Low to moderate amounts of oils and good fats (ideally plant based)
- Sweet, bitter, and astringent tastes
- A mix of dense, heavy, or creamy and occasional clear, cleansing foods
- Most green veggies
- Coconut or sweet fruits for snacks

Avoid:
- Salty, spicy, sour, or acidic foods
- Hot foods and substances
- Oily foods and substances (like fried food, fatty meats, avocado, nuts, and seeds)
- Meat intake, especially darker meats and salty meats and seafood

Herbs/Spices

Most kitchen spices are not beneficial for pitta because they are heating in nature, but there are a few exceptions:

- Coriander (which is the seed of the cilantro plant)
- Mint
- Saffron

Women with high pitta can explore herbs and substances that act as gentle laxatives:

- Raisins
- Aloe vera
- Rose
- Amalaki

Cooling herb tonics can also be used:

- Hibiscus
- Neem
- Sandalwood
- Shatavari

Herbs and spices can be taken in room-temperature or slightly warm water or milk. Cow, goat, sheep, oat, or coconut milks are often soothing and cooling substances for pitta.

SLEEP

Develop a regular sleep routine with a set bedtime that you follow every night. Pitta-dominant people tend to burn the midnight oil because they are doers, but they often crash very hard. Go to bed earlier than you are inclined to, preferably by 10 PM, and if you are not tired yet, spend time winding down until you can relax and let go.

EXERCISE

Practice slower and cooling types of exercise — either first thing in the morning or later in the day. Gentle walks are good, as are gentle yoga and tai chi. These activities may feel a little slow and boring, but they are exactly what the pitta-imbalanced individual needs. Swimming is another great exercise for pitta. Do not choose workouts that are very intense, because pitta is already hot and inflamed. On the other hand, do not choose anything that bores you too much, because you won't stick with it! Balance happens incrementally — it's not binary. You don't necessarily have to quit the things you love to do, but you need to learn how to do them more sustainably — slowly and with less intensity.

MIND-BODY PRACTICES

Pitta-dominant people often have the easiest time meditating because they are good at concentrating. They can benefit from meditation that opens their awareness, given that their minds can be too narrowly focused — even on tasks and ideas that are not helpful or healthy — because they can become addicted to accomplishment and reaching conclusions. Any type of meditation that broadens awareness and creates slowness can be beneficial, such as body- or sensory-scanning exercises and a meditation focused on letting thoughts go.

Pitta-imbalanced individuals can also benefit from cooling breathing exercises, such as *sheetali pranayama*. To practice sheetali, curl your tongue in from the sides so it looks like a little straw (if you have a body that allows you to do this tongue position!). Breathe in through the little straw, feeling the cool air on the tongue, and then exhale out the nose, feeling the cool tongue press into the sinus cavity and spread coolness the head. Continue breathing in through the tongue as a straw and exhaling out the nose, as you gradually begin to feel the coolness spread all over your body.

Limit breathing exercises that are fast or intense, such as *kapalabhati pranayama*, because they typically create more heat.

BODY TREATMENTS

Reducing inflammation is important with pitta imbalances. Treat the part of the body that is inflamed with cooling substances. If there is an inflamed joint, applying cooling ghee or coconut oil to the skin will help soothe it. If there is a red rash or acne on the skin, apply cooling, anti-inflammatory cilantro or aloe vera juice for a few minutes and then rinse with lukewarm water. Neem is also wonderful for inflammation issues. Be gentle with pitta imbalances, because roughness and rubbing will make them worse. Sometimes the best medicine for pitta is to simply leave it alone, rather than trying to correct the imbalance. A reactive body can start to react even to things that are normally helpful. Also, choose skin products that do not contain a lot of oil if you are already very oily.

Pitta dominance can make you susceptible to irritation in both the skin (external and internal) and the eyes. Taking a lukewarm bath with mint leaves, mint essential oil, or rose petals can be very soothing and cooling. Soaking in a cool pool, relaxing in a sensory-deprivation tank, getting gentle body treatments, or wearing an eye mask to block out light is helpful to soothe irritation. Pitta eyes can be relieved by using eye drops infused with rose petals.

The most effective body-balancing treatments for pitta involve taking laxatives to purge heat from the liver and sometimes reducing blood volume through giving blood. Many women with pitta imbalances notice that they feel remarkably better during their period — like an overall body release is happening. A pitta-dominant woman may need more release than others, and it's possible to get it through some of the herbs noted below.

SEXUAL PRACTICES

Healthy sex includes having healthy tissues afterward. Because pitta-dominant individuals can become inflamed easily, moderation is the key for sex. Having sex once a day, a couple times a week, is likely well tolerated by a pitta body. However, having sex multiple times in one day or every day can cause vaginal and cervical inflammation. It's good to give the body a rest for a day or two so any minor pitta imbalances caused by sex can rebalance. If there is more intense inflammation, then it can be helpful to take a couple of weeks to rest before having sex again.

Pitta-Balancing Daily Routine

Pitta-imbalanced individuals tend to ignore all advice they do not agree with and implement perfectly the advice they do agree with — sometimes *too* perfectly. Therefore, a pitta woman is encouraged to take on a little bit less than she is inclined to.

So, a pitta-pacifying sample daily routine might look like the following.

PITTA-BALANCING DAILY SCHEDULE

TIME	ACTIVITY
6:30 AM	Waking up
6:45 AM	Drinking a cup of lukewarm mint tea "Letting go of thoughts" meditation 15 minutes of tai chi
7:15 AM	Shower
8:00 AM	Breakfast
11:00 AM	Drinking a cup of warm milk with saffron and rose powder
1:00 PM	Lunch
3:00 PM	Drinking a cup of warm water with one half teaspoon of amalaki
6:00 PM	Dinner
9:00 PM	Lying down and doing gentle yoga while listening to soothing music
10:00 PM	Bedtime

If you suspect a pitta imbalance, factor in your existing daily routines and sketch out a new, ideal schedule that will help slow and cool things. Think about creating spaciousness and softness and putting less effort into things. Make sure to note regular activities, including items like recurring meetings and repeating activity times. Sometimes, for a pitta person, simply adding a chunk of time into the day with no agenda and no commitments is hugely impactful.

How realistic does this feel to you? Pitta-imbalanced individuals benefit by adding spaciousness and slowness and reducing busyness and ambition, so sometimes the best medicine for pitta is allowing yourself to be a little more of a slacker.

Sensory Superpowers of the Fertile Years

The menstrual cycle alters your state of being — both physically and mentally. Most women know all the things they hate about their menstrual cycle — the cramps, headaches, bloating, and moodiness — but few real-ize that there are actually some superpowers that also come with having a menstrual cycle. A woman who is really tuned in to her body might notice these, while many others might not even realize they are present!

It's really about perspective. Many women feel more sensitive during certain phases of the cycle and may find themselves annoyed with some-thing in their environment. However, are they also noticing that those same sensitivities are increasing pleasure from other things in the environment?

The way we experience the world is through our five senses, and one of the key components of a balanced body is having a balanced relation-ship with these senses. We need the senses to perceive what is in our envi-ronment, to make good decisions, and even to enjoy beauty. On the other hand, if we are too involved in the senses, the world can sometimes seem like it's filled with extreme amounts of pleasure and pain, which can then become a distraction to peace. And, if one sense becomes blocked or cut off, sometimes the experience of another becomes stronger. The latter phenomenon is one of the drivers behind closing your eyes in meditation.

There is no doubt that the senses are important. We need them. Taste and smell both give us clues about the nourishment we need. Imagine being a chef without being able to taste or smell food. Imagine if you were a musician and could not hear.

For a woman, her senses sometimes shift during the course of her cycle. For example, many women report feeling a heightened sense of smell around ovulation (referred to as lower olfactory threshold) or being more sensitive to noise in the days before menstruation begins. Partially, this is because of shifts in body awareness as we change physiologically throughout the month, but there may also be some biological purpose underlying these shifts. For example, if you catch a whiff of an attractive manly smell, then maybe that will stimulate the desire to have sex! Also, sensitivity to noise might give you more desire to be alone and in a quiet, restful place, which isn't a bad thing if you are just about to get your pe-riod! Once you start paying attention to these superpowers, you will never look at your cycle the same again.

As with all sensory processing, three main parts are involved in perception: first is the object being sensed; second is the sense organ detecting the object, plus the associated peripheral neuroanatomy involved in relaying the sensory information to the central nervous system; and third is how the central nervous system interprets this information. Sensory processing is affected not only by the condition of the inbound channels but also by the mind. Any pain we experience may be an issue with the body being overly sensitized to a certain quality or could be an issue with the mind's processing of the sensory input, and oftentimes it is both. Remember, the urges of your body trump your mental urges when you are tapping into your primal self. Pay attention to even the weird sensations of the body — even if they don't seem to make sense, and even if they spoil your plans. Listen to what the mind says, but trust the body more.

The five senses are associated with certain sense organs on the body. Sound is captured in the ear, touch on the skin, sight in the eyes, taste on the tongue, and smell in the nose. Understanding that inbound sensations may become more sensitive at certain times of the month is helpful, as is studying any pain or discomfort that recurs with each month's cycle, because these patterns can give clues into the types of doshic imbalances occurring in the body.

Sound and touch are associated with vata, sight with pitta, and taste and smell with kapha. An individual with high vata may have a very sensitive body and tolerate only gentle massage. A high-pitta body may have sight issues. A high-kapha person may have a lot of nasal congestion.

Vata-imbalanced people may have more difficulty at the start of the period, pitta people during the middle-to-late phase of the cycle, and kapha people just after the period ends.

The relational superpower of vata is detachment. Pitta's is persuasion, and kapha's is loyalty. All such qualities can be perceived as either negative or positive, so when evaluating Ayurvedically, it is most important to see how these doshas are affecting the physiology and quality of tissues.

Recognizing and Addressing Kapha Dominance

Oh, kapha-imbalanced individuals, in some ways you have it the easiest, and in others you have it the hardest: easiest because kapha-imbalanced people often have more of a sense of calm; and hardest because their conditions can be some of the most difficult to reverse. Signs of a kapha imbalance include slowness; excess wetness; sliminess; heaviness; lethargy; a tendency to gain and hold on to body mass more easily; longer menstrual cycles; and tissue growths, like tumors, cysts, or warts. Kapha-imbalanced individuals typically sleep well, and often sleep too much.

General Signs of a Kapha Imbalance

- Lethargy, heaviness, or moving slowly
- Excessive sleep
- Wet respiratory system — sinus, throat, and lungs
- Excessive urination or water retention
- Tendency to gain and hold on to body mass more easily
- Tumors (including fibroids), cysts, warts, skin tags, or other growths
- Excess hair growth
- Congested digestion — nausea, constant sense of fullness, or mucus in stool
- Longer/slower menstrual cycles
- Sweet or fishy smell to the breath or body

If you've been experiencing signs of a kapha imbalance, then you can follow the kapha-dominant preconception rituals. Excess wetness or earthiness can slow down information transfer, which means that a kapha body takes longer to react than other bodies. Kapha bodies can also have reduced space due to the excess water, as well as tissue growths that can block channels and tubes, so a kapha imbalance must be taken seriously if you're preparing for conception. Kapha bodies are often the least receptive, and if there are metabolic issues resulting in toxic ama formation, then this makes conception even more difficult.

The kapha-reducing rituals involve warming and drying the body, creating a roughening effect on the imbalanced tissues, creating space, and breaking down any overgrowths. Kapha is a "building" state, and as mentioned earlier, a pregnant body is also in a building state. Removing tissue growths and excess dampness from the body before getting pregnant is beneficial for your health and will improve your chances of conception. It's important to try to correct a kapha imbalance beforehand. You will not be able to reduce a kapha imbalance much during pregnancy, since building energy is needed for the baby, and the two of you will be sharing a blood supply, nutrition, and other vital fluids. If you are not able to shift a kapha imbalance prior to conception, then you will have to wait until after the baby is born and possibly until after breastfeeding is complete, since you will need lots of moisture to create breast milk.

The qualities of kapha are *cool, wet, heavy, dull, slimy, static, dense,* and *cloudy*. Are any of these qualities feeling all too common for you? Do you note any of these in your physiological functioning?

To balance kapha, we must open ourselves to some discomfort in how we interact with the world — because kapha requires measures that are *asantarpana*, or not nourishing. The goal is to increase heat and movement, break down tissues, and dry out the body more. Basically, kapha requires what some would view as tough love, but it may not actually feel like a bad thing, because kapha-dominant people are generally less sensitive. Having a more receptive body and increased energy is likely to feel amazing.

Kapha is protective, lubricating, and stabilizing. A woman's kapha increases just after menstruation ends, and while she is pregnant to support the rapid growth and changes that are to occur. However, in excess, kapha can create stagnation, blockages, and growths.

Examples of excess kapha in the reproductive tract are cystic conditions of the ovaries or uterus, fibroid tumors, uterine polyps, or mucus in the period blood. Reproductive systems with mildly high kapha have slower menstrual cycles and will menstruate less frequently, since the body does not heat up as quickly, which sometimes means that a woman with this type of body will be fertile for a longer duration than other women simply because she's had fewer menstrual cycles in her life and lower levels of tissue degeneration. However, kapha imbalances mixed with toxic ama can create blockages in the system, which lead to abnormal tissue development in the form of growths and ultimately interfere with the menstrual cycle and fertility. The bottom line is that while kapha is protective, it can also cause disease if it's present in excess, especially if the metabolism, or agni, is compromised.

SIGNS OF A HIGH-KAPHA REPRODUCTIVE SYSTEM

- Later menarche
- Less frequent cycles
- Longer menstruation duration — bleeding for many days with moderate amounts of blood
- Little body-temperature spike during ovulation
- Mucus or chunky matter present in menstrual blood
- Reproductive-tissue growths — cysts, tumors (including fibroids), or warts
- Fertility into older age
- Excess vaginal fluid and discharge
- Heaviness in the pelvis or low-back stiffness before menstruation
- Feelings of attachment, greed, or sadness
- Disinterest in sex (due to complacency)

A woman needs kapha for sex to be functional and painless. If she has low kapha, the vagina will not be lubricated (a vata condition), sex will become painful, and she may as a result start to have signs of inflammation or burning (high pitta). If she is not biologically aroused for whatever reason (work stress, life stage, systemic imbalance, or lack of attachment to her partner, to name a few), then having sex is not recommended, because it will injure her body. Kapha increases with attachment and will keep the body lubricated. A woman will crave sweet or sour foods when her body needs more kapha to perform a function.

Because conception requires ample space — space for the ovum and sperm to travel through, and space for a baby to grow in — high-kapha situations should be taken seriously if a woman is preparing for pregnancy, because they take up that space and block connection. Interestingly, the emotions associated with attachment, like sadness and greed, are linked to high kapha, so it is important for them to pass through and be cleared from the body. Even becoming overly attached to a partner you love, a family member, a pet, or your own child can prove to be not so great for your health, if it increases kapha too much. The key is finding the space between too much and not enough.

Menstrual fluid that contains mucus is the water aspect of kapha, and the cycle between periods may be a little longer because a lot of water in the body can prolong the buildup toward ovulation and delay it, as water takes time to heat up. Water helps mix things and provides lubrication against roughening actions.

The earth element is also an aspect of kapha. Too much earth creates fibroids, cysts, and polyps. A period with too much earth may have chunks of membranes or other solid pieces in the menstrual fluid. Too much earth gives one the sense of heaviness and downward-moving energy. Too little earth would result in very short periods, due to thin uterine lining. A baby needs earth stable enough to hold on to but not so dense that it cannot implant itself to receive nourishment.

The following section includes dietary and lifestyle recommendations for a woman with a kapha imbalance, plus recommendations for mind-body practices, body treatments, and helpful herbs.

Kapha-Balancing Dietary and Lifestyle Practices

BALANCING QUALITIES TO EXPLORE

Hot, dry, clear, subtle, mobile, rough, and dispersing

DIET

Eat no more frequently than every 5–6 hours, and not when you aren't hungry. Kapha bodies naturally stay in building and maintaining mode longer, so they tend to have the weakest appetites, simply because their bodies do not break down or metabolize as quickly. Their bodies will turn all metabolized matter into something they hang on to for a while. Eat only when hungry to avoid toxicity, congestion, and metabolic issues.

Favor:
- Eating less frequently
- Heating and drying foods, including spicy foods
- Pungent, bitter, and astringent tastes
- Light, clear, and cleansing foods
- Smaller meals
- Roughening foods, like raw salads, popcorn, and other drying foods
- Hot, liquid foods that can move stagnant energy

Avoid:
- Sweet, salty, or sour foods
- Sweet or sour fruit
- Cold, creamy, or dense foods and substances, including most dairy
- Oily foods and substances (like fried food, fatty meats, and nuts)
- Meat and seafood intake

HERBS/SPICES

Kapha types benefit from many spices in the kitchen, since most are heating and drying, including:

- Pepper — black as well as spicier types
- Thyme
- Rosemary
- Clove
- Oregano
- Basil
- Garlic powder
- Paprika
- Turmeric
- Ginger
- Cardamom
- Mustard seed
- Marjoram
- Sage

Women with high kapha can explore medicinal herbs that act as warming, stimulating, scraping, tightening, or fluid-moving agents, such as:

- Bibhitaki
- Camphor
- Chitrak
- Manjistha
- Punarnava
- Guggulu

Herbs and spices for kapha conditions can be taken with hot water and honey, which is a heating and scraping substance.

SLEEP

Kapha-dominant individuals typically do not have trouble getting to sleep or staying asleep. On the contrary — they need to make sure they are not getting too *much* sleep. Too much sleep will make it even more difficult to get moving and motivated, and it's challenging to decrease the water and earth elements when you aren't motivated to move. If you are dealing with excess kapha, and are used to going to bed early, then try waking up an hour earlier in the morning so you can exercise.

EXERCISE

Get up early and do a little bit of exercise as frequently as you can, ideally every day. Twenty minutes of vigorous exercise each morning will melt, spread, and cleanse the excess wetness and earthiness from the body. Try running, cycling, *vinyasa yoga* (also hot yoga), dancing, or some other type of exercise that will make you sweat. Choose practices, teachers, and even music that have the qualities of being light, fast, hot, and motivating. Focus on quick, dynamic movements, rather than holding positions for a long time.

MIND-BODY PRACTICES

Kapha-dominant people should spend time meditating, moving, and breathing. They have the most patience to sit for a long period of time, but they need to move more than they sit. Kapha-imbalanced individuals are typically calmer and less reactive under pressure, so they may need stress-management techniques less than other people and would be better off spending their time focusing on desires, goals, and affirmations.

An individual with excess kapha would benefit tremendously by practicing a variety of yoga breathing exercises. Kapha-dominant people can try most breathing exercises, including fast and intense ones that can be drying for others. *Ujjayi* and *kapalabhati* are the best breathing exercises for a body with excess kapha because they are energizing and warming, and can help cleanse out the excess mucus from the respiratory tract.

Ujjayi pranayama, meaning "victorious breath," is a common type of breathing practiced in some popular yoga classes today. First, inhale through the nose and then exhale slowly. If you pretend you are fogging up a mirror on the exhale, you are constricting your glottis in your throat, and if you close your mouth while constricting the glottis, your breathing will sound a bit like Darth Vader. Continue to breathe in and out through the nose, making your Darth Vader noise as you exhale with the mouth closed. Take full, long breaths. Repeat for 10 breaths, and continue with 1 or 2 more rounds if you like.

Kapalabhati pranayama means "skull-shining breath." To practice it, take a breath and exhale most of the air from the lungs; then right before the end, quickly force the rest of the air out via a sharp, focused exhale. Let the inhale happen naturally and then force the next exhale out quickly, and repeat. The breaths are shallow and rapid, rather than deep. Imagine that if you held a feather in front of your nose, you would be making it jump with each exhale. Essentially you are repeating a short, shallow exhale, and the inhale happens automatically. Repeat for 30 breaths and then pause. You may stop after this round, or practice 2 more rounds of 30. As you become more adept at this breathing exercise, you can increase the number of breaths per round, but do not go too quickly. Allow yourself at least a few days to practice the number you are on and see how it affects your body, mind, and energy before you make a move to increase it.

BODY TREATMENTS

Kapha-dominant bodies are tough. They can tolerate a bit of roughening, like deep-tissue massage, dry brushing, and other exfoliation methods. In fact, these are very beneficial, because kapha bodies do not break down and regenerate as quickly as others, and their fluids need to be encouraged to move so they do not stay stagnant. They can also tolerate dry saunas and visiting the desert more than other constitutional types. Getting fluids to move and clear out is a balancer for kapha, so sweating techniques — especially dry ones — are helpful.

Oils and oil massage are not recommended for an issue related to kapha, a dosha that is already moist and grounded. The exception is a massage with mustard oil, which is very heating. Inhaling the aromas of certain essential oils, such as camphor, clove, and cinnamon, can also be warming and stimulating.

The most effective body-balancing treatments for kapha involve sweating, roughening, and lightening. Reducing swelling in the body typically enlivens kapha, and the swelling can be discharged through sweating and excretions. Some individuals with kapha imbalances experience a natural urge to vomit, and this should never be held back (other natural urges, like sneezing, urinating, defecating, flatulence, and yawning, also should never be held in, or they cause physiological issues). Vomiting is a way for the body to quickly remove excess fluids, as is diarrhea, sweating, and urination. If the focus is on discerning what behaviors and conditions led to the queasiness, then a kapha imbalance can actually be prevented.

High-kapha conditions can tolerate and even benefit from the aroma of brewed coffee and the smoke of heating and drying herbs, such as sage, clove, or rosemary.

SEXUAL PRACTICES

Kapha-dominant people are generally blessed with lots of juiciness and have great endurance. Therefore, not only can they typically have more sex than others, but it can actually be good for them to do so, because it helps move the excess vital fluids in their bodies and can be stimulating and cleansing. On the other hand, kapha-dominant individuals may be a little slow to gain an appetite for sex, because complacency is one of the traits of excess kapha.

Kapha-Balancing Daily Routine

Kapha-imbalanced individuals are slow to get started, but once something sticks, it sticks. Therefore, a kapha-dominant woman may need a little bit of coaching when beginning preconception practices. And then, once therapeutic measures are implemented, she must be on the lookout for when it's time to end them, since her routines are often hard to break.

So, a kapha-balancing sample daily routine might look like the following.

KAPHA-BALANCING DAILY SCHEDULE

TIME	ACTIVITY
6:00 AM	Waking up
6:15 AM	Drinking a cup of hot water with black pepper, ginger, turmeric, and honey 5 minutes of ujjayi or kapalabhati pranayama 30–60 minutes of jogging, cardio, dance, or a dynamic, warming yoga practice
7:15 AM	Shower
11:00 AM	Brunch
3:00 PM	5 minutes of ujjayi or kapalabhati pranayama or a brisk walk outside
6:00 PM	Dinner
10:00 PM	Bedtime

If you suspect a kapha imbalance, factor in your existing daily routines and sketch out an ideal sequence of activities that will help quicken your pace and heat things up. Be sure to build in time for doing something new and energizing, such as the breathing practices described in this section, or some other enlivening pursuit or practice you enjoy.

Are you feeling motivated? Push yourself to get a little less comfortable than you are inclined to, and if you are having trouble getting motivated, that is all the more reason to hire a practitioner to help you over the hump of starting out.

Multiple Doshas at Work?

It is important to note that some conditions actually involve two or more doshas, so it's a bit more complex. Also, you may have different types of imbalances in different parts of the body, though people typically have one or two dominant imbalance types. Nevertheless, this should give you an understanding of how the different qualities of the doshas affect a person in general, and specifically affect the reproductive tissues. Now you can start reading the tea leaves of your body, and you have some basic protocols to address imbalances.

Reproductive Agni

So how do you know if the agni (metabolic fire) of the reproductive tract is in balance? First, it is important that the main digestive fire be balanced and that an individual eat according to the strength of this fire, since it is the root of most diseases. Changes made on a macro level with the digestive tract can affect the tissues of the reproductive system. Second, you can tune in to your cycles — understanding what is normal and healthy for your body — and begin to study the biological cues that this system sends you regularly.

Each cell and tissue type has its own form of agni, as discussed previously, and the reproductive system is diverse, so it involves multiple forms of agni. The muscles have agni, and the muscles of the uterus are responsible for contraction and movement of materials in or out of the reproductive tract. The blood has agni, and since the blood's role is to bring energy and nutrition to vital systems of the body, including the reproductive area, the blood agni governs the delivery of energy. Even the fluids of your body have agni — kapha makes up the plasma part of the blood, as well as the lymphatic, interstitial, and other lubricating and mixing fluids. You've probably heard the saying "Where your attention goes, energy flows." The body follows this rule, but we also need to add that energy goes where it's free to move. It flows as long as it's not blocked.

Each tissue type, or *dhatu*, whether functioning as a solid or liquid, has an agni that can be balanced, too weak, too strong, or erratic in some way. Below are the main types of tissues in the body, according to how Ayurveda views it. These tissues contain cellular structures, air, water, nutrients, and so forth, but they are bound by a common purpose that makes them function similarly.

DHATUS OF THE BODY

TISSUE TYPE	FUNCTION (DRIVER OF AGNI)
Plasma	Providing lubrication and mixing
Blood	Delivering energy and nutrients
Muscle	Facilitating action
Fat	Providing protection
Bone	Providing structure
Marrow + nerve	Filling spaces and moving energy
Reproductive material	Supporting procreation

Healthy reproductive functioning is a sign that the overall immunity and stamina of the body is strong. The reproductive dhatus of the body, *shukra* and *artava*, are the last to get nourishment, so if a person is depleted overall, then the materials that would be used for creation will also get depleted. Shukra is the male semen, which contains sperm, and artava is the female menstrual fluids that the ovum is released into and/or washed out of the body with. Both shukra and artava have their own agni, and this has an impact on fertility. The seeds inside the shukra and artava may someday be used for a new body altogether.

One may notice patterns between aspects of the reproductive

tissue and the rest of the body. Sometimes a whole tissue type can get affected in several sites in the body, such as what can happen with low muscle mass. A woman may have reduced muscle in her arms and legs (a sign of high vata), and her uterus may also be very thin or small. Conversely, women with larger muscles naturally may find themselves with a thicker uterus. Women who significantly lack fat on their bodies might encounter nerve-related reproductive issues because of a depleted myelin sheath (the fatty covering around nerves) and also experience anxiety or problems with memory from reduced fatty tissue in the brain. These women may not menstruate, because oftentimes the lack of fat results in an overall reduction of kapha dosha, and when there is not enough nourishment and water available, artava dhatu gets depleted and reproductive functioning suffers.

Cells also have their own form of desire, and they, too, can get damaged if their agni is imbalanced — either too weak or too strong. If a cell is weak or defective in some way, especially if it's still getting a lot of energy, it is more likely to become affected by a dosha when an imbalance occurs. As stated earlier in this chapter, weak spots are vulnerable, and when the body gets out of balance, it's often these weak spots that suffer the most.

Six Types of Therapeutic Measures in Ayurvedic Treatments

Many people are curious about what Ayurvedic treatments entail. The truth is that as an ancient medical system that individuals are still practicing today, Ayurveda offers innumerable possibilities. However, each type of treatment, whether it uses traditional methods or modern advancements, can be categorized as having one of six different types of effects on the body.

1. **Langhana,** or lightening therapy, would be involved when there are issues of heaviness, clogging, density, and blockages.

Examples of these types of therapies are fasting and exercise that lightens the body. Langhana is used for conditions with ama or high kapha.

2. **Brahmana,** or building therapy, would be used when a person needs stability or mass. Examples of these types of therapies are eating nourishing and building foods, practicing stabilizing exercise, and using certain medicinal oils externally or internally to strengthen the tissues. Brahmana is used for conditions with high vata.

3. **Swedana,** or sweating therapy, is used when a person needs to reduce the water element, eliminate toxins through the sweat glands, or deliver herbal medicines in the bloodstream to the skin area. Examples of these types of therapies are taking a dry or wet sauna, exercising to the point of sweating, or taking medicines to increase sweating. Swedana is used for ama, as well as various vata, pitta, and kapha conditions.

4. **Rukshana,** or roughening therapy, can be used to scrape or agitate tissues to unblock channels and encourage movement. Examples of rukshana therapies are dry brushing, exfoliating, brushing your teeth, or eating "roughage." Rukshana is beneficial for conditions with ama or high kapha.

5. **Snehana,** or oleation therapy, would be administered on someone as a protective measure or as a preparatory measure for other therapies that may involve movement or agitation. Examples of oleation are performing an oil massage, drinking oils, and administering nasal oiling. Snehana is beneficial for vata and some pitta conditions, and any condition in which ama will be cleansed from the body.

6. **Stambhana,** or tightening therapy, can be used to reduce the size of a channel and to stop fluids from leaking from the body. Examples of stambhana therapies are drinking astringent herbs or teas and applying tightening masks to penetrate

the skin. Stambhana is beneficial for reducing the space element inside a channel and for stopping excess secretions from pitta or kapha.

You must keep in mind the end goal, because these therapeutic measures can backfire when not applied skillfully. The duration and magnitude of therapy, as well as the order in which each one is delivered, are very important. Context is key. I mention them here for your consideration so that you get a conceptual picture of what an Ayurvedic professional might teach you to do for yourself. These measures can be carried out via body treatments, herbal remedies, dietary measures, exercise practices, and so forth.

Make Healing a Priority

If you want to have a child and are dealing with some imbalances in your body and mind, then can you work on this before you conceive? Life gets more complicated and the body goes through major changes after conception and birth. You are not truly healed until you fully understand symptoms and their causes. This requires you to educate yourself about how bodies generally work and how yours works specifically. You need to study your thoughts, actions, and environment and see how all these things affect your body. This is an ongoing process. We should be getting wiser as we get older, but if we neglect our issues, this will not happen. Make self-study your continuous priority and real learning will take place.

All you have to do is try your best. You don't have to torture yourself. Everything you do to make healthier choices is valuable and absolutely worth it, even if things don't feel perfect. I'm hoping that learning about Ayurveda has given you a new lens through which to view how your body and mind work, and that this makes balancing your health a more intuitive effort for you. If you have ama, metabolic toxicity, then you should focus first on cleansing before you undertake these healing therapies.

Read your physical, mental, and emotional signs and see if they match up with any doshas you observe in your cycle. Look for signs of ama toxicity — blockages, coating, plaques, or areas you can't feel. With this information, you take steps going forward to remove toxic blockages and balance the doshas, working with a professional as necessary.

Chapter 9

Your Partner

You make love differently to women
of delicate or rough temperaments.

— **WENDY DONIGER**, *Redeeming the Kamasutra*

A woman can expend energy prepping her own body and mind for conception, but it takes two to tango. A woman's natural fertility journey has one other very special person involved in the process: her male partner. Whether it's her husband, her boyfriend, some guy she met at a bar one night, or a donor dad, chemistry matters. A man's physiology has to function properly, too, in order for him to produce and deliver good-quality seeds for a new life. Even more importantly, the more she comes in contact with this partner, the more the two of them will influence each other's health. Their energies, and even their fluids and their cells, mix and affect each other's physiology. If we follow the principle of *like increases like, and opposites balance each other*, then it becomes evident that the qualities of the individuals we have relationships with can influence our state. In addition, any imbalances affecting one person can also affect the other. The integrity of our individuality is maintained by being a unique and vibrant human being, which Ayurveda says happens when we have good-quality tissues; balance the doshas, agni, and mind; and are abiding in our own nature.

Physiology, body chemistry, and a little bit of the mysterious cosmic power of the universe are what make a baby. Therefore, it's important for your partner to be healthy so that he is also more fertile. Even beyond fertility, though, you and your partner need to be healthy so that the two of you can live well together — regardless of whether a child is in your life. Just as *you* will want to be on firm footing when you conceive, with your best health and in a healthy environment, your partner will also want to be in good position. Everything the two of you do to be vibrant, healthy, passionate, and in a safe and supportive environment will be beneficial for you and your future child.

Fertility requires the reproductive channels of the man and the woman to be healthy, and this is supported by the overall health of the body. This isn't just about sex — it's also about making sure the parts involved in sex are open channels. Infertility can be due to a problem on either side and in some cases both. Therefore, it's equally important that the woman *and* the man care for their health.

Men also have a kind of biological clock, but their fertility doesn't "run out" as quickly as a woman's. They can produce sperm for decades longer than a woman can ovulate, with minimal disruption to their bodies — whereas for women, it becomes a safety challenge to grow and birth a baby in an aging body. However, the quality of a man's sperm changes and degrades as he ages. Kapha and pitta decrease in older age, and vata increases. As vata increases, a man's juiciness also declines — plus, his sperm count, mobility, and motility are affected by degeneration. He is subject to the same laws of nature that all humans are, though his parts operate a little differently from a woman's.

So, is there any way to know ahead of time that you and your partner can have a natural conception? This chapter attempts to give you a few tools to scope out his health and how it affects your.

Understanding Your Partner's Vitality

Intimate relationships require tremendous vulnerability but also tremendous strength. It's sometimes difficult to determine true compatibility — because, on the one hand, there is what the mind wants, and sometimes the body signals that it wants something else. On top of this, our desires can be fleeting, so how can we trust that we are really on the right track with a potential partner?

A woman can use Ayurveda to choose the best partner; understand his vitality; and improve their relationship physically, mentally, emotionally, and spiritually. Whatever bodily imbalances she has going on inside her will color her mental, physical, and emotional experience of the world. This can actually happen so pathologically that sometimes a person can create false realities and fail to see situations for what they truly are.

Take, for example, a pitta-imbalanced woman who is dealing with issues of intensity, inflammation, quickness to judge, and constant transformation — she may always be hypercritical in relationships. She can feel like her life, or the life of her partner, is never good enough. Her relentless obsession with perfection can ultimately sabotage her ability to experience joy in her day-to-day life. And sometimes it can spill out and affect her ability to form a long-term intimate relationship. The longer-term problem with not balancing the pitta dosha is that this same energy can shift into hypercritical thoughts about colleagues, about not being a good enough mother or her partner not being a good enough father, and maybe, at a certain point, about the child not being good enough in some way. However, if she balances the pitta inside her, then she may be able to slow things down, cool off, and enjoy the moment more.

Similarly, a woman with a vata imbalance will come to the table with more fear or anxiety, and she may feel that her partner is causing it at times. Because *like increases like*, our relationships certainly affect us, but we should be working to keep ourselves balanced in the process. If she balances her vata, then she will be able to tolerate more of the qualities that can cause imbalances of vata — mobility, chaos, uncertainty, quickness, subtlety, spaciousness, and the like.

Learning to see ourselves and our partners clearly is a key skill that will help us become better parents. Each of us has a mental, physical, emotional, and energetic dimension. We must get to know our own dimensions, and through our relationship with our partner, we can also get to know a bit about his dimensions. I learned at some point that I could never know what is going on inside my partner's mind unless he told me, despite the stories I often told myself about him. Even if we try to explain another person's behaviors, we can base our explanations only on limited information. It is always best to learn about the mental and emotional dimensions of our partner based on his own feedback, because there is only so much we can read into.

The Four Fertility Factors — *seed*, *season*, *field*, and *water* — also apply to men. Through learning about Ayurveda, you'll recognize some observable details that can give you a clue about what is going on within another person's body, which can be helpful when trying to understand your partner's experience and vitality. For example, men have their life seasons, and their environment and lifestyle also affect their physiology and reproductive strength. Men are not always used to sharing their emotions, but often you may get insights into your partner's emotional status if you can read the doshas objectively. If you have clues, then you can ask skillful questions to get to know your partner's thoughts and feelings more deeply.

For instance, if you notice that your partner is having trouble sleeping and is constipated, you might assume that vata is at play, and you can ask something like, "How long has your health been feeling disrupted?" If you notice that this always happens to your partner when he has a big work meeting coming up, then you might be able to bring up that pattern as a discussion point.

Studying a person's body is a doorway to deeper knowing, but we cannot make assumptions about the contents of another's mind — the mind is much more unpredictable. The best we can do on our own is projection — thinking of how we would be feeling in that person's situation based on our own life experience and biases — but projection is not actually understanding how that person really thinks and feels. For that, we need feedback.

Your Partner's Physical Body

Just as studying your body is important, studying your partner's physiology and constitutional type is very telling, as is noticing the quality of his excretions and his energy. When the doshas are imbalanced in a man, they generally give signs similar to those that occur in a woman. Factors such as body composition, amount of saliva in the mouth, condition of skin, body odor, and elimination patterns can give clues about a man's doshas as well.

Here's how you can use your senses to better understand your partner's physical layer.

PERCEIVING DOSHAS THROUGH YOUR SENSES

SENSE	VATA	PITTA	KAPHA
Hearing	Dry, scratchy, raspy, higher-pitched voice or quick speech; anxiety, fear, or worry connoted in words; noisy digestive system due to gas; body cracks and pops	Sharp and penetrating voice; criticism, anger, or aggressiveness connoted in words	Deep voice or slow speech; stubbornness, attachment, or excessive calmness connoted in words
Touch	Dry, cold, rough skin; quick, thin, or snaking pulse	Hot, moist skin; strongly thumping pulse	Cool, moist skin; slow or thick pulse
Sight	Dry-looking skin or a darkened tint; jumpy eyes; brittle or frizzy hair; minimal sweat	Red or ruddy skin; penetrating eyes; fine and oily hair, baldness, or early gray; frequent sweat	Pale and juicy-looking skin; big and soft eyes; thick and plentiful hair; excessive sweat upon exertion
Taste	Mouth or body without any taste	Salty, pungent, or sour-tasting mouth or body	Sweet-tasting mouth or body
Smell	Mouth or body without smell	Pungent or foul-smelling mouth or body	Sweet- or fishy-smelling mouth or body

If you can get your partner to share information about his wastes and excretions with you, then you can also do the same sort of analyses you do on yourself — studying urine, stool, and sweating patterns. Some couples don't feel comfortable sharing this information with each other, but it's really helpful if you do and can actually end up being a surprisingly fun bonding experience.

Does your partner seem tired and lethargic, overly animated, or fairly level? Is he consistent, or is his energy erratic? Have you noticed anything about his breathing?

A man's breath energy, or *prana*, will affect people around him. His prana will be influenced by his diet, his exercise routines, and other lifestyle factors. The goal is not to have high prana. The goal is to have balanced prana. Even too much energy can be a problem. Prana is the subtle essence of vata, so with too much vata, oftentimes prana can also be raised.

A man's heat and light energy, or *tejas*, will affect his glow and sense of passion. It, too, will be affected by diet, exercise, and other lifestyle factors and routines. Having balanced tejas is important. Tejas is the subtle essence of pitta, and we've all gathered that too much fire burns.

A man's stamina is *ojas*, which is also often correlated with immunity. Being the product of good nutrition and healthy agni, a man blessed with ojas will have the ability to endure and withstand illness. Ojas is the subtle essence of kapha, so with too little ojas, one's immunity suffers due to lack of protection. With too much, one's immunity can also suffer due to blockages being created.

The development of healthy tissues requires balanced prana, tejas, and ojas. These subtle energies are the essence of the gross energies of vata, pitta, and kapha. Balance in these areas will create healthy immunity, energy, and drive.

Your Partner's Mental State

Remember in chapter 2, where I introduced the two minds a woman has — the intellectual and the primal? Well, a man has these two minds, too. At any given moment, a man is also mostly being dominated by his primal or subconscious self, while the intellectual or conscious mind, with its discernment and its rational thoughts, plans, and ideas, seems to give everyone the impression that it's in charge. This is good to know, because if your man can seem confusing to you sometimes, then you might be a little more forgiving. It's a lifelong study for us to know ourselves! It's good for you as a partner to see if what a man says and does are aligned, but it's even better if he has also evaluated himself emotionally and physically, because it's a deeper way of knowing one-self. Knowing one's heart, mind, and body leads to the strongest integrity in a person.

Just as a woman may be confused about what she wants and feels, so may a man. Fears, insecurities, irritabilities, and resistances are all possibilities when the mind gets involved. Therefore, it's important for the man to be in touch with his primal body, too. You may share what you've learned with him and maybe even some of the same question-naires that you filled out earlier in the book, but he may get inspired by another way to tap into the primal, which is also very good. The most important thing is curiosity about oneself. It can help to be using the same frameworks to evaluate your health, but as long as you continue to try to observe, listen, and understand each other, you can both come from different places and still find ways to connect and relate.

In summary, we experience other people physically, energetically, and mentally. How we feel when we are around a person matters tremendously. We feel their heartbeats, taste and smell their bodies, see their behaviors, and hear their voices. Our direct perception of their qualities will raise those qualities in us. Then we take this sensory information and start mixing it with what's already in our minds — memory, beliefs, or expectations. This causes us to have certain mental or emotional reactions. Any emotion we feel — anger, fear, attachment, and even the feelings we associate with love — facilitates a tangible, physiological response in the body. Therefore, it's not only our direct perception of a person's qualities that affects us but also the qualities that get activated from our own memory and life history. This is how even thoughts can contribute to an imbalanced dosha! The good news is that the mental layer can be one of our most changeable layers.

Whenever any of us feel out of balance, we have to study what it was that caused us to get in such a state in the first place. That is the only way we get at the root cause of illness and prevent disease. Was it something in the environment that caused us to go out of balance, or was it perhaps our own errors and misperceptions?

Self-Reflection in Relationships

One of the reasons why meditation is helpful for a lot of people is because it's an opportunity for self-reflection. Meditation allows you to watch your thought mechanisms, improve them, and eventually let go of them so you can have clear, direct perception. When you have clear, direct perception, you can trust your intellect to make good decisions. If you are distracted, it's difficult to truly trust yourself. When you can trust yourself, you will choose the right partner and make generally healthy relationship and life choices.

Writing is another way of self-reflecting, because you literally get to see your thoughts. Jot down for yourself any observations you've made about how your partner affects you — physically, mentally, emotionally, and energetically. Also note anything about your partner that you are currently emotionally charged or confused about. Make a plan to discuss these current emotions with your partner and try to understand both your own feelings and his side of the story. Ask yourself, *Are these emotions limited to my relationship with my partner, or do I feel them in other relationships, too?*

Next, write down some of what you've discovered about yourself — good or bad! — since you've started this relationship: thought patterns, behaviors, desires, fears, and so on. It's interesting to think about the things you like and dislike about your partner, but it's far more impactful to think about the things you are learning about yourself.

The more challenges you go through with another person, the more you will learn about yourself in the relationship. This doesn't mean you should seek a partner who is difficult to get along with or stay with such a person, but every relationship is an opportunity to learn about all the dimensions of yourself. It's how you resolve the challenges you both face that will bring you closer together or further away from each other, physically, mentally, emotionally, and energetically.

Promoting Male Fertility

Fertility involves all layers of a person. Your partner should aim to be healthy in every one of these layers — for himself, and also so that the quality of his sperm is good. As with women, men can be provided with fertility-promoting rasayanas: a diet and lifestyle protocol, plus spices, herbs, and body treatments, based on their constitutional type and life circumstances. In addition to balancing the doshas and agni — and cleansing, if necessary — Ayurveda also uses *vajikarana*, or the discipline of promoting or enhancing fertility in a depleted person.

You are probably aware that the culture that brought us the first work of literature on sexual methodology is the very same one that brought Ayurveda and yoga to the planet. Early on, the Vedic culture could see that sex was the source of both tremendous pleasure and also challenges and suffering at times. The *Kama-sutra* is believed to have been written on the Indian subcontinent about 200 BCE, around the same time that the first Ayurvedic medical text, *Charaka-samhita*, was written. While the *Kama-sutra* discusses numerous methods for sexual intercourse, the Ayurvedic texts, like the *Charaka-samhita* and the *Ashtanga Hrdayam*, discuss sex from more of a health perspective, outlining ways to promote sexual energy and develop both healthy reproductive tissue and healthy seed. (Unfortunately, the level of detail on women's reproductive health in these classical texts is quite limited compared with the attention given to men's. That is not surprising, since all the texts were written by men.)

A Man's Seeds

A man's body can seem a little less mysterious than a woman's because his main reproductive parts are visible from the outside. However, there's still a lot going on inside that will affect his fertility and sexual functioning. The scrotum alone has more than just two little egg-shaped containers in it. It's actually the center for the creation, maturation, and storage of sperm cells.

Starting inside the testicles, cells and chambers are responsible for the creation of male seeds — germ cells, or *spermatogonia*. This first step in generating sperm starts at puberty for a male, whereas you may remember from earlier in this book that a female's germ cells are created in utero. These germ cells are the seeds that ultimately morph into the sperm. The testicles also hold the channels and junctions where these male germ cells turn into more mature male reproductive cells. The testes have several tissue types, including skin, nerves, muscles, blood vessels, and connective tissue, and house channels that move the sperm cells along through a process called peristalsis, which is a wavelike muscle contraction that moves objects and fluids through a channel. This just so happens to be the same type of wavelike motion that functions to move food through the digestive tract. Peristalsis is vata in action.

Sperm are matured, protected, and fed before they are released to the world. Incubating sperm have very sensitive temperature requirements. There are actually little muscles that pull the testicles up close to the body when they need to be warmer and other muscles that lower the testicles to cool them. After leaving the testicles, the sperm sit in a storage area also inside the scrotum, called the *epididymis*, where they are well nourished before being released out of the body via ejaculation through the urethra's opening at the end of the penis. On the way out, other organs secrete fluids that help the sperm swim, providing nourishment, protection, and lubrication to mix with a woman's fluids should they meet. The sperm, like the ovum, needs an open channel through which to pass, so once again healthy tissues are important.

If you look at a sperm under a microscope, you can see that it is a living organism. It has unique parts and looks like some sort of microscopic tadpole. It can live on its own for a while, and it can penetrate through cells like a needle delivering a vaccine, based on its own actions. A woman's ovum, on the other hand, is passive. It is carried from the ovary, down the fallopian tube, and later into the uterus by wavelike motions of fluids and structures of the reproductive organs.

The egg is static. The sperm is mobile. Which has the more difficult job — the one having to do all the action or the one having to surrender to its environment?

Balancing Sexual Energy

The reason why we should care at all about mastering our sexual energy is because it's so pleasurable, and pleasure is tricky for humans to deal with. When we experience it, we want it more. Sometimes we seek pleasure so much that it takes us over and clouds our ability to reason. Power is reclaimed when we see our pleasure mechanisms and decide whether we are going to allow them to rule us. A self-realized person can see her own cravings and determine if they are appropriate for her biological requirements and life circumstance — evidence that the primal and the intellectual are on the same page.

Another reason to master one's sexual energy is because the timing of sexual arousal can be an issue for some people. For many men, it seems that they want sex all the time, and for others, maintaining an erection can be difficult. Sexual arousal and activity is influenced by both physiology and psychology. The penis has the ability to fill with blood very quickly and also to be emptied of that blood quickly. In a healthy man, who is well nourished and has balanced agni, doshas, and mind, the desire to procreate is a natural one. The same goes for a woman, though her urge gets influenced a little more by the fluctuations of her menstrual cycle. When a man or a woman has lost sexual desire, both the body and mind are factors.

Sex is truly a magical act. It's what creates new people. It's magical and it's also sacred. You are allowed to enjoy it when the urges arise, and at the same time, you need to make sure you do not become so narrowly focused on these urges that you cause issues in either body or mind. If a woman pays attention to her body, mind, and menstrual cycles, she will develop clarity and balance in her relationship with sex. Likewise, a man can study his own body, mind, urges, and semen to balance *his* sexual energy.

A man's semen tells a lot. His diet and lifestyle, climate/seasonal factors, and his life stage will all affect how his doshas are present in

the semen. Healthy semen is "thick, sweet, unctuous, without any pu-
trid smell, heavy, viscid, white in color, and abundant in quantity." Vata
sperm is dry and scanty. Pitta sperm is runny and has a yellowish tint.
Kapha sperm is plentiful, thick, cloudy, and dense.

Men are more often virile in their younger years because they naturally have more kapha dosha in that phase of life. As the body is met
with the intensity and stress of middle age, kapha declines some, and
then as a man dries out in older age, the kapha and pitta decline more.
A man who has a vata-dominant body type may lose his virility earlier
than a man who is pitta or kapha dominant. Well-nourished men, who
have balanced agni, are the most virile.

Male Reproductive Issues

Just as a woman's reproductive issues can be balanced once the telltale
signs of dosha imbalances or ama toxicity are understood, so can a
man's. The markers are just a little different. Here are some examples
of common male reproductive issues, plus treatments to balance overall body and sexual energy and create healthy tissues, according to the
type of imbalance.

DEALING WITH MALE REPRODUCTIVE ISSUES

MALE REPRODUCTIVE ISSUE(S)	POSSIBLE CAUSE(S)	TREATMENTS
Dry or scanty semen; low mobility or motility of sperm; low sperm count; premature ejaculation	Vata imbalance	Balance vata: More water, oil, and nourishing foods in the diet — even meat — with warming spices and seasonings. Bone broths from domestic, wetland, and aquatic animals are recommended. No raw or dry foods. More rest, slowing down, and staying warm. Less frequent sex so that fluids can be replenished.

MALE REPRODUCTIVE ISSUE(S)	POSSIBLE CAUSE(S)	TREATMENTS
Yellow-colored semen	Pitta imbalance	Balance pitta: Fewer heating foods and activities. No meat. Favoring sweet, bitter, cooling foods. Slowing down and reducing effort. Regulating sex to prevent inflammation and rehydrating with cow or coconut milk afterward.
Excessively thick and cloudy semen	Kapha imbalance	Balance kapha: A reduced quantity of food or less frequent eating. Favoring heating, lightening foods and spices that spread or dissipate moisture and enhance movement. Activity. Having lots of sex.
Low sex drive; difficulty maintaining erection	Ama toxicity blocking the reproductive channels; circulation issues due to vata and/or kapha imbalance; being in the habit of not having sex; mental disturbances	Strategically cleansing and then rejuvenating with vajikarana therapy (see below).

Vajikarana Therapy

Vajikarana is an ancient Ayurvedic therapy focused on increasing quality and number of sperm, desire, and the strength and luster of the body — and creating healthy babies through contentment with sex. Vajikarana is not necessary if an individual already has a healthy sex drive and healthy sperm, tissues, and so forth. As with all Ayurvedic therapies, treatment is necessary only when there is an imbalance. You must know the type of imbalance before treatment. Ayurveda is concerned with making sure there is proper nourishment and care for a body that may lose some of its fluids and cells through sex. In addition, it assumes that low sex drive during the prime fertile years of life is a sign of an imbalance. On the other hand, too much sex depletes semen and sperm, reduces strength and immunity, and raises vata in men. Depleted semen can also be caused by the wrong diet or lifestyle routines, compromised agni, stress, emotional issues, disease, or even repression of natural urges like urinating. The goal is to find the balance point between biology and desire, because this leaves a person healthy overall.

The main characteristics of vajikarana treatments include those qualities that will increase both agni and kapha. Examples of these qualities are:

- Passion
- Attachment
- Nourishment
- Unctuousness
- Sliminess
- Earthiness
- Sweetness
- Saltiness
- Sourness
- Heaviness
- Routines

A person can add such qualities to the diet and environment. Interestingly, kapha can become depleted by too much heat, but in vajikarana treatment, the objective is to give the heating foods along with the moistness and heaviness of kapha-building foods. This allows them to harmoniously work together to replenish tissues.

Ayurvedic texts actually say that the best motivator for a man's sexual energy is "a sexually excited female partner," so while it may be interesting to focus on balancing your man's energy, it's even more important for you to focus on balancing your own sexual energy. If a man is unable to rejuvenate his sexual energy through diet and being around a sexually excited partner, he may try cleansing and then taking the herb shilajit orally, or he can try a dashmool herbal enema or sesame-oil enema for added therapeutic benefit, provided his colon is free from signs of inflammation or injury.

Ayurvedic treatment always aims to get at the cause, rather than simply delivering relief of symptoms. A person's body must already be properly cleansed internally before any vajikarana treatments are given. This is because if you provide extra nourishment on top of an existing imbalance with any ama/toxicity mixed in, the treatment will be unsuccessful. A channel has to be prepped and cleansed strategically first. Like rasayana, vajikarana is the rejuvenating therapy given after cleansing. My feeling is that cleansing is a delicate process better managed with the help of a trained Ayurvedic professional, because if it's done improperly, it can make conditions worse.

A Complicated Relationship with Sex

If you have ever evaluated your overall relationship with sex, as I did when I started thinking about becoming pregnant, it can be very confusing. First of all, I was raised Catholic, so that alone gave me a weird relationship with sex. Then, when I started to get into Indian philosophy, I could see that some of its works were obsessed with pleasure, some with health, and some were interested in doing weird things with one's body. I felt a lot of conflict inside about sex, and no reasonable advice seemed to be offered by any of my teachers or the "great books" they studied.

I remember sitting in yoga teacher training in the middle of the rainy Costa Rican jungle one afternoon, and the teacher asked us to translate the word *brahmacharya*, and then comment on it. You could feel everyone start squirming in their seats. *Brahmacharya* means "holding back one's sexual energy." All of a sudden, yoga teacher training started to feel a bit like going to my teenage catechism classes. All the conflicting feelings I had about sexuality seemed to rise to the surface. Was sex evil, and a sin, or was I just like any other animal?

I immediately became defensive. I liked sex. I didn't want someone turning me into a monk, especially since I wanted to have kids someday. On the other hand, I could tell that my relationship with sex was not always healthy. I'd let my desire drive me to make poor decisions on many occasions. At times, I'd failed to respect myself as much as I could have, and even felt that others did not respect me enough. As I studied yoga longer, this word, *brahmacharya*, always came back to haunt me. I already felt some sort of Catholic guilt about sex. Why did these ancient and modern yogis want to rub salt into my wound?

When I led yoga teacher trainings later on, I started to teach other yoga teachers about this word that gave me such mixed feelings. It was always tricky to talk about with people. Ironically, I've always learned more by teaching than I have by studying. Through discussion with my students, I realized that *brahmacharya* means different things to different people, because everyone has a different relationship with sex, and it changes throughout a person's life. A monk takes a vow of celibacy so that he or she can achieve certain spiritual states, but this doesn't mean he or she is healthier than others (look at what happens with Catholic priests). A person who is interested in becoming a mother naturally, on the other hand, actually needs to surrender to her sexual urges, because those are the ones that create a baby! Therefore brahmacharya is not an either-or, yes-or-no thing. It's basically a dial that has strength at different degrees, depending on circumstance and intention.

The wisest thing to do is to develop a balanced biological relationship with sex. Everything else we might think about sex due to our religious backgrounds, relationship histories, and expectations of what it's supposed to be is just mental chatter that we need to let go of. We want our reproductive tissues and organs healthy, so having sex at a frequency that feels healthy for our bodies is important. Sex drive changes based on health, monthly cycle fluctuations, life stage, and mental-emotional factors. We want to remain strong and vital, so we don't partake excessively in sex, the same way we don't run a marathon or eat a box of chocolates every day. We must mentally maintain power over our desires so that we can always make the best decisions.

Sexual energy is powerful. We use it to fuel creative endeavors. How we wield this energy is personal, and it's a practice. This energy creates people, so brahmacharya is perhaps one of *the* most powerful yogic practices out there.

Developing Connectedness

Life is just a collection of moments, and in order for you and your partner to have a life together, you must jointly experience the same space and time. Repeated rituals build routines, such as eating dinner together or going out on a date every Sunday. Rituals practiced as a celebration of the past or to draw attention to a special intention for the future bring with them the energy of inspiration and affection. Birthdays, weddings, and holidays are examples of such rituals. Maybe the two of you even want to create your own special preconception ritual as you set off on this journey together.

Because a relationship is complex, and ebbs and flows with the physical, emotional, and mental state of each person in it, it's also important to focus on building connectedness within your partnership. It's possible for two people to live a life together side by side — sleeping in the same bed and eating dinner at the same table every night — without truly connecting. It's even possible for two people to have sex and not feel connected with each other. However, once a little intention is placed on a true connection, everything can change — and it's worth it.

You cannot assume that your partner will always feel the same way you do, but you can work on your own sense of connectedness. You must have your own practice in place to cultivate this. When you're connected, *you* will be a better partner. When your partner is connected, *he* will be a better partner.

In my own self-discovery process, I realized that I can easily connect with mental and physical constructs, but when it comes to my heart space, I have challenges. Talking with clients, friends, and family members, I've seen that we all experience this at times. If you find yourself in a similar place, then chapter 6 may be a helpful one to revisit, because the practices can assist you in refocusing your intention — and there you will rediscover your heart.

Speaking of chapter 6, if your partner is open, you can each add something to your ritual space that signifies your intentions together going forward and that even serves as a preconception ritual the two of you can share. Or it could be that the act of getting married or moving in together is the stating of intention, and the ongoing relationship is a commitment to that original intention.

Everyone has their own way of tapping into intention, and what works for you may not work for your partner. My own partner may see me meditating, sitting in front of one of my sacred objects at home, or hear me chanting to some deity that inspires me, but he doesn't participate. My practice is not something he can relate to, but I suspect he appreciates what I do because it makes me happier.

> *Let the beauty we love be what we do.*
> *There are hundreds of ways to kneel and kiss the ground.*
>
> — RUMI

There are so many different ways that people tap into their deepest hearts. Find yours and love it. Feel free to express it to your partner, invite him into your inspirational rituals and activities, but do not expect him to have the same methods. He has to find his own way in, but you will inspire him with your bright light.

Chapter 10

Your Environment

And every breath we drew was Hallelujah.
— LEONARD COHEN, "Hallelujah"

As discussed earlier, the Four Fertility Factors are *seed, season, field,* and *water.* When we talk about the field, we are referring to the space surrounding the baby and everything inside it. First and foremost, you are the closest field for the baby, because your body supports the egg and because later you gestate, give birth to, and breastfeed the baby. Your partner is at the center of the field, too, since he provides the sperm to activate this potential new life and define its characteristics, plus he cares for both you and the baby. Your job, leisure activities, house, and city, as well as where you travel to, are also in the field. The field is everywhere you and your partner go, everything you both eat and take in with your senses, and everyone you both interact with. It includes your biology and mind, along with the social network, family, and community environment that surround you, the seed, the fetus, and then the growing baby.

The environment surrounding you, your partner, and the baby will bring out certain aspects of your psychology and biology. The place where a woman lives, the people she is around, and the nourishment in her environment all influence her biological rhythms and how her body and mind respond to stimuli. She, in turn, influences her macrocosm, and then by choosing certain environments, she influences her microcosm.

The diagram below shows the field from the perspective of the baby being at the center and everything around the baby being inside it:

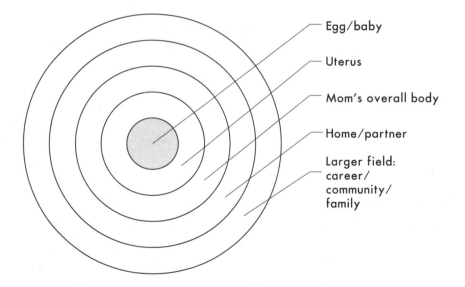

Egg/baby

Uterus

Mom's overall body

Home/partner

Larger field: career/ community/ family

Figure 6: The "field" surrounding the egg

It's important to assemble your personal field in the way that suits your life as closely as possible. You haven't met your child yet, so you aren't really sure what that child will need, and it's best to focus on your own needs. Yes, I said *focus on your own needs*. To start, simply look at your own body in your present-day life and environment. If your body and mind are somehow out of balance, then you have your answer, and now you must determine the changes necessary to find homeostasis. You can utilize the Ayurvedic tools in previous chapters to perform this body- and mind-rebalancing work, but there are also times when you have to make decisions about your broader environment, because the sounds, sights, smells, textures, and tastes you come in contact with — like the food you eat — influence your health.

Later, you may apply what you've learned from Ayurveda to reading your baby's health if you are tasked with that.

You Come First

You may remember in chapter 4 when we discussed that the field, or kshetra, is a place where a person may take a pilgrimage. A baby would certainly be embarking on a pilgrimage, but you yourself are also on a great pilgrimage. All life is special and sacred — and yours is the main one you can try to direct the course of.

Your goal as a woman considering having a child is to place yourself in environments conducive to your own good health. Your partner needs you healthy. A baby needs you healthy. In addition, you make the best decisions when you are healthy and your mind is sattvic — whether it's choosing a partner, job, where to live, or what to eat for lunch.

Here is the priority order: (1) you, (2) everything else. You've probably heard a flight attendant on a plane tell you that even if you are traveling with children, you have to put your own oxygen mask on first in the event of an emergency. Your health helps everyone else in your life. When you are not healthy, it isn't good for anyone around you, either.

Most of this book has been focused on how to get your body healthy so that you bring your best physiology and tissues to the table in your life and for conception when the environment is right. You can employ the self-care tactics I outlined earlier. They will help. I've also discussed your partner's role, and hopefully you've gotten some insight about his vitality and how important it is to note how you feel inside when you are around him. However, shifting into a broader focus on the environment surrounding you may also be very helpful.

Aligning the Inner and Outer Worlds

Your life is a collection of experiences, decisions, and actions that un-fold in various environments. If you read your environment well, make sound decisions, and take action with integrity, you are more likely to have thriving health. To read your environment well, you need aware-ness, and this awareness is of two kinds: internal and external. Internal awareness is the experience of your body, mind, energy, and memories. External awareness is of the environment, whether it's home, work, or somewhere you have traveled to. You have the ability to sense your en-vironment and also how it makes you feel inside. You process what you perceive, and then take action.

The ability to discern between something beneficial (*hita*) and harmful (*ahita*) is a necessary life skill, but this can be challenging at times because it can often be difficult to identify the cause or root of a problem. We may spend time blaming something in our environment for hurting us instead of looking at the things we are doing to hurt ourselves. What makes matters worse is that sometimes our minds and senses are not clear. Clarity is not a bunch of mind chatter. Without a clear mind, we cannot have accurate perception, and when we do not have this, we cannot trust ourselves.

If both mind and body are doing objectively well, then you are in good stead, but if something is off, you need to pay attention. Even if you are experiencing something physical, your senses and/or mind may be corrupted somehow and clouding your perception. The knowl-edge of the body trumps everything else, because it's physical proof of what's happening. If you are off, then you have to start comparing your thoughts, actions, and feelings with what you are seeing happen in your body. You may not be giving your body what it needs to operate optimally, or something in your environment may be harmful to you. Note: in both of these scenarios, you are in the driver's seat. You can't blame the environment — you have to change how you interact with it by making different choices. You can try to effect a change in your en-vironment, but if this does not work, then your health may fare better if you move to a new one.

Checking In with Your Environment

You need to find the positions in your life where your good juju can shine through. Place yourself in environments that you thrive in — around plants, people who inspire you, structures that support you, and so forth. Let others rely on you. You will feel useful and connected. Don't seek environments where you feel the life being sucked out of you. Don't go where you do not feel safe. Don't go where you lose your self-control. Go where your body operates well and your mind and senses are clear.

Let's look at where you are spending your time. It can make all the difference.

Home Field

This sounds like some sort of baseball reference, but what we're talking about here is the environment in which you live — your abode. The home field is wherever you spend your most intimate time, doing the types of tasks that you repeat every day, like eating, sleeping, showering, engaging in leisure activities, or cuddling up with your partner. Whether you own a home, rent an apartment, or live in a room in your parents' house, the space you are in has certain qualities that affect you. Your job is to try to influence the environment to make it comfortable and beautiful. The trick is knowing how to design for this.

The people in your home and the furniture, artwork, plants, music, smells, space, and amount of sunlight at certain times of the day all affect your state of being. If you live in an apartment building, your neighbors affect you, too, due to their proximity. A soft bed will increase kapha, lowering pitta and vata. Having no air-conditioning or fan in a room will increase pitta during a hot summer. Light-colored walls create a sense of spaciousness, and cooling colors are cooling to the body. Plants pacify pitta. Water pacifies vata. Having animals generally increases kapha, though each animal also has its own doshas. Every detail matters in your environment, because it reinforces certain qualities in you.

I had a client suffering from a vata issue that would get worse whenever she got busy, mobile, or unsettled. She was working really hard, meeting with a lot of clients, and traveling a lot due to a long-distance relationship. Her life had gotten so out of control that she couldn't implement changes in her daytime activities, so we focused on the only downtime she had — sleeping. Turns out, she was sleeping on an air mattress, and by the middle of the night, it would lose all the air and she would end up freezing on a cold, hard floor. She was going to be moving soon, so she didn't want to invest in a new bed. When I pointed out how the bed was contributing to her vata imbalance, she said, "Oh my god. You are so right! I totally fantasized about crawling into my roommate's bed last night." She then borrowed a thick futon from a friend until the big move.

Whenever we feel that something is impermanent, it raises vata. Even though we know nothing is permanent, it is helpful to trick our bodies into believing otherwise sometimes — particularly in those moments when we do not feel settled. This is where the power of rituals and affirmations come in.

Sometimes when a woman is living with a partner, she feels that he is negatively affecting her. I've had many women ask me how to deal with their partners' imbalances. This is a challenge because sometimes there really is an issue with the partner, sometimes there's an issue with the woman, and oftentimes both. When this happens, I advise my clients to focus on balancing themselves, first and foremost. If a woman takes the actions necessary to create more health and balance in *her* life, she should theoretically improve the lives of the people around her, too. If she feels better and then those around her do not, it becomes clear that something is going on with them. Remember, we have to put on our own masks first. Then we can be of some value to others.

The Larger Field

These days, it seems the world has gone crazy. We are exposed to so much sensory stimulation — both positive and negative — and it can become very overwhelming to deal with it all. We may cope by retreating, reacting, or behaving in a way that dulls our senses. The sensory input, and the overwhelm we feel from it, affects us on a mental, physical, and energetic level, so it must be addressed.

In my thirties, I went through a period when I didn't read or watch the news for a few years. This was during the time of my life when I meditated every day for thirty minutes religiously — for six years. I had already gotten rid of my TV and it was before I had a smartphone, so I wasn't really on social media that much, either. I heard the news through my friends. It was an interesting time because my worldview could have become highly influenced by everyone around me, but I was meditating so much, that didn't happen. What I started to notice was how differently people reported on what was going on in the world. Everyone seemed concerned with different issues. Some of my friends were concerned about politics, some about how the food and agricultural systems were being run, and others about the performance of sports teams or the lack of females in corporate executive positions. I asked myself, *Why do people care about these things, while I am happy sitting in my apartment writing?*

There is an entire smorgasbord of happenings and information out there that people can get concerned about, but due to all the meditation I was doing, I was so internally focused that somehow I didn't care about any of it. It felt freeing, mentally and emotionally. At the same time, people close to me would become angry with me for not getting upset about certain things going on with the world. I didn't hate the same companies they hated. I didn't really care about the local sports team. In all my internal contentedness, I also started to have a difficult time relating to people, because they were so wrapped up in these happenings.

But there were other things I did care about, and people I could relate to on those levels began to enter my life. I cared about becoming a mother, so my life became filled with people who seemed supportive of that journey. I cared about self-development, and I had lots of people in my life who were engaged in various flavors of it. I cared about writing, so I joined a poetry group and I even hired a writing coach.

A lot of my female clients find themselves in a place where they don't feel they fit well with their current environment any longer. This is one reason why retreats are so helpful. I know that when I went off to the Costa Rican jungle to do my first yoga teacher training, I really wanted a break from my life, or maybe even a restart button. When I came back, my meditation practice became a way for me to keep having this break from life. However, constantly needing breaks from life is not only inefficient but also not sustainable when you have real-life demands placed on you. What I really needed was to learn how to *be* in my life without getting myself into a place where I felt like I needed a break from it.

Humans project our inner state onto the outer state. Whenever I see problems with the outer world, I know that there is some problem inside me that I am trying to sort out, too. When I get those mental urges to revolutionize the environment around me, what I really want is to revolutionize something within myself. When I see everyone around me as toxic, I look for the toxicity in me. When I balance myself, I am my best version of *me*, and the world is better.

Helpful Environmental Changes

The environment around us will always be changing, and the only thing we have to do is read it, while also reading ourselves, and that is how we stay truly healthy. Sometimes environmental changes actually help us healthwise.

Can you think of a time in your life when you had an issue that was suddenly resolved because the environment changed? You went to Hawaii and your dry skin got better. The neighbor moved and you could sleep better. The rainy season ended and you stopped feeling sick and tired all the time. It could even be that your favorite brand of ice cream was no longer sold in the store and you were forced to pick a snack that wasn't such a metabolism killer.

Paying Attention to Environmental Shifts

Can you think of anything in your current environment — at work, at home, or during leisure activities — that seems to be causing you any stress or ill health? Next, focus on some environmental changes that seem to be helping your health. As the environment around you shifts — whether it's seasonal changes or something going on in your relationships — your doshas can change, too.

One way to improve accountability when you want to rebalance a pattern is to note when changes in your environment will make a change in yourself easier. This is one way to learn how to tap into nature's rhythms. Otherwise, it can feel like trying to swim upstream when the current is simply too powerful to fight against.

Our memories can be very short — we can feel that we were good one day because we didn't eat cake, but we forget the next and go right back into eating cake every day until we start to feel lethargic. We forget that we set an intention to be on a better path. This is why, when we want to change something, it actually takes time to get reprogrammed. The hamster wheel we are on is powerful.

If pitta is imbalanced and you are going into summer, which is pitta season, then you may need to work that much harder to balance it. If the water element is too high and you are in the middle of rainy season, then your drying actions have to be that much stronger. Similarly, if vata is already high as you are going into fall, be prepared to ground, warm, and nourish yourself.

Designing Sensory Input

Another way to make your changes stick better is to bring reinforcements into your environment. Everything that comes in contact with your five senses has the ability to influence your state. Sensory input will affect physiology and even trigger certain memories.

Therefore, you can influence your internal state by designing the environment to increase or decrease certain qualities.

Influencing the Senses

Remember from earlier in the book, we learned that like qualities increase like qualities and opposite qualities balance each other. The gunas, or attributes, are shifting from environment to environment, person to person, season to season, and food to food. This all happens within the field. You experience the field through your senses and what you eat. You influence the field based on your mind and your actions.

You can use the senses to balance the qualities you are experiencing.

You have five of them to play with. For example: If you feel hot, expose yourself to cooling tastes, smells, and feeling sensations. If you feel like things are moving too fast, listen to music with a slower tempo. Here are some more examples of how this works:

WAYS TO BALANCE THE SENSES

SENSE	EXAMPLES OF BALANCING ACTIONS
Hearing with ears	To reduce slowness, play fast music To reduce lightness, play deeper tones To reduce dryness, play water sounds
Feeling with skin/body	To reduce roughness, apply smooth substances To reduce coolness, take a hot bath To reduce sharpness, wear soft fabrics
Seeing with eyes	To reduce dryness, apply water- or oil-based eye drops To reduce mobility, stare at a fixed object, such as a lit candle To reduce heat, surround yourself with more pastel green and blue colors
Tasting with tongue	To reduce density, eat foods that are porous or full of air To reduce cloudiness, eat clear foods To reduce heaviness, try eating lighter or less food or fasting
Smelling with nose	To reduce wetness, sniff drying scents, like clove and camphor To reduce heat/inflammation, sniff cooling scents, like rose and jasmine To reduce subtlety, smell anything strong!

Playing with the senses is how we artfully balance body and mind in Ayurveda. It's how we make choices to bring in slightly different sensory input. Next, we'll go a little deeper into how the taste of food affects us.

The Six Tastes

Your digestive tract is part of your field, your environment, since each of its organs are hollow spaces inside you. How you process your food may be similar to how you process the space around your body. There are six categories of taste, and each of them affects the mind and body differently. Women can artfully direct nourishment of the body by playing with the tastes, textures, timing, quantity, and combinations of foods. This artful play with the body's input, and the study of its output, is a skill that comes in extremely handy when a woman is learning about her own reproductive health and, later, the health of her baby.

Your kitchen is healing when you make the right foods and drinks for your constitution. Even restaurants and cafés can be healing, but you need to know how to order for your constitution. (Have I told you I don't really like to cook that much? I'm sort of a master of Ayurvedic ordering of restaurant food.) Cooking at home gives you more control.

You can use the six tastes to create certain effects in your body. When you know the effects that each taste has physiologically and energetically, you can become a little more strategic in how you eat. Here's the gist of how the six tastes affect your body.

THE PHYSIOLOGICAL EFFECTS OF THE SIX TASTES

TASTE	ELEMENTS INCREASED	EFFECT
Sweet	Water + earth	Sweet taste is cooling, builds tissues, and creates more water in the channels of the body. You will find the sweet taste in most baked goods, sweet fruits, many grains, and anything with sugar.
Salty	Water + fire	Salty taste increases heat in the body and creates water retention and sometimes inflammation. You will find the salty taste in meats, cheeses, saltwater fish, and anything with added salt, including most prepackaged and processed foods.
Sour	Fire + earth	Sour taste increases heat and heaviness in the body. It causes downward secretion of fluids. You will find the sour taste in citrus, yogurt, tomatoes, tamarind, kombucha, and papaya.
Pungent	Air + fire	Pungent taste increases heat and upward-moving air in the body. You will find the pungent taste in ginger, garlic, raw onion, and any type of pepper — the hotter the pepper, the more powerful, generally.

THE PHYSIOLOGICAL EFFECTS OF THE SIX TASTES
(CONTINUED)

TASTE	ELEMENTS INCREASED	EFFECT
Bitter	Space + air	Bitter taste is cooling and causes movement and spasms in the body. You will find the bitter taste in most green leafy veggies and also in beer and black coffee. (This is one reason why coffee makes you run to the bathroom. So do other bitter things.)
Astringent	Air + earth	Astringent taste is drying and tightens tissues. You will find the astringent taste in black tea, alcohol, spinach, and beans.

Let's explore some examples. If you're trying to speed up metabolism, then the tastes that facilitate heat and/or movement are key: pungent, bitter, salty, and sour. If you're trying to reduce inflammation, then cutting down on salty, sour, and pungent foods can help, but if you're trying to increase the water element, then sweet and salty foods are the way to go.

All substances we ingest may have one or more tastes, so it can get a little confusing. One food can have multiple medicinal effects, so you have to discern which are the most powerful in any given mixture.

How to Eat Ayurvedically

Contrary to what you may have heard about Ayurveda, there is no such thing as Ayurvedic food. Many people call food Ayurvedic if it's Indian because Ayurveda originated in India, but actually any food can be Ayurvedic. It has to do more with the qualities of the food and the context in which it is consumed, and less with the actual ingredients used. This is a delicate nuance but an important one, because if you start thinking that all foods or even products labeled Ayurvedic are good for you, you are getting yourself into the same thought processes that wreck everyone's health in the first place — that is, focusing on labels and ideas as gospel, while not paying attention to the context of life in front of you right now.

There are foods used a lot in Ayurvedic medicine, though, because they've been tested on body types extensively. For example, kitcheree (also spelled "kitchari" or "khichdi") — which is typically a porridge of rice, mung beans, oil or ghee, and spices — is often used in Ayurvedic healing fasts because it's a very simple, tridoshic (that is, applicable to all three doshas) recipe that most people with gut issues can digest and that can be altered easily to suit a person's health demands. However, let's look a little closer at a non-Indian food: hummus. It's made up of garbanzo beans (also called chickpeas), which are astringent and raise vata. It's also made up of lemon, which raises kapha. It's got some salt, garlic, tahini (sesame-seed butter), and maybe even some olive oil, and all those raise pitta.

Now, the main ingredient in hummus is garbanzo beans. Beans are drying, so we can assume that hummus will principally raise vata. Lo and behold, hummus also gives a lot of people gas, which is one purvarupa (early symptom) of excess vata conditions! Therefore, if you are a vata-imbalanced person eating hummus every day in vata season, which is fall, you're just going to raise vata more if this consumption is not reduced or countered with a balancing substance, such as olive oil. Then you may wonder why you're having anxiety, difficulty sleeping, and muscle spasms, but it doesn't have to be a mystery anymore if you learn about Ayurveda.

Ayurveda is about applying principles to how you eat. It's not about eating Indian food. This is important to understand, and hopefully it makes your Ayurvedic journey more practical and fun. It did for me. While I really enjoy Indian food, there are a lot of other foods I like more. (Italian is my favorite. Note that marinara sauce is really great for vata but not so great for pitta and kapha. Everything has a time and a place.)

The macrocosm affects the microcosm, and vice versa. You need to design both your micro-field inside you and the macro-field around you for optimal health and fertility. What you do internally will affect your external world. What you do externally will affect your internal world.

Designing for Beauty

Beauty is a balanced, inspired, and connected state. Beauty is not an object, but there can be beauty within an object. It may be in the relationships you are forming in your life; in your home or work environment; or even in something as trivial as your clothing, jewelry, or lipstick.

When we feel something is beautiful, this happens because it has qualities we want more of. When we feel something is ugly, it has qualities we want less of. In a discerning person, the judgments of what is beautiful will be beneficial to health.

Some women wear makeup because they want to accentuate a part of their bodies that they think is beautiful. Other women wear makeup because they want to hide something they don't feel good about. Do you see the difference? True beauty allows more beauty to come through. It doesn't allow hiding and shame to clog up pores further. Beauty is inspiring.

Take a moment to contemplate the beauty that already exists in your life. Where and how do you feel beauty when you are at home? What about at work? Are there special objects that evoke a sensation of beauty within you, whether they are on your body or in your environment for you to see?

You are in a beautiful time of life. Take time to recognize where beauty already exists. Keep beauty as your friend. Inspire yourself and others in your environment.

Conclusion

How to Be Healthy and Fertile

You've read the book, so let's recap what we covered. We went over the basics of health and fertility according to Ayurveda and the challenges that modern life presents for women to align with nature. We covered ways for you to overcome these challenges. You've learned more about yourself. You've contemplated your larger life and also your partner's health. You've started experimenting with the ways you can carry your intentions into your everyday life. Hopefully you are developing some consistency.

This last section is intended to be a quick reference for you to brush up on the core ideas of the book. Please reread this section from time to time to reinforce your learning and intentions. You can even share it with your partner and others in your life who are supporting you on your journey. Reading these pages will allow your partner to get involved in your fertility journey without having to read the whole book himself, though he might be interested in chapter 9, "Your Partner," as well.

Preserving Your Health and Fertility

I want to leave you with one simple idea: the best thing you can do to preserve your fertility and overall health is to surrender to nature. The more you try to avoid, control, or outsmart it, the more you will get in the way of its work. Now that you know the Four Fertility Factors, you can settle into the wisdom of your body a little more. As you understand and then learn to surrender more to the urges of your body, you will simultaneously create the best conditions for conception and the environment to support the growth of new life.

Let me summarize a few key rules to live by that we covered in this book to help you align with nature. Just do your best with these and don't worry about the outcome:

1. Know that your desire to have a baby is not what will get you pregnant; the desire to have sex is what will.
2. Learn to spot vata, the energy that governs movement; pitta, the energy that governs transformation; and kapha, the energy that governs stability.
3. Look at your poop, pee, emotions, and menstrual blood regularly to understand your doshas.
4. Balance your doshas to the optimal levels for your body to function well — not too much or too little.
5. Remember that your agni, or digestive fire, is your body's true hunger and passion for life, and learn to understand the difference between appetite and true hunger.
6. To correct an imbalance of one quality, add more of its opposite quality.
7. If something in your environment is toxic, reduce the amount of it in your life.

8. Cleanse before you try to conceive if you have a lot of toxicity or experience blockages to pregnancy, and don't forget to rejuvenate after the cleanse, because that's just as important.

9. Let your emotions inform you; they are a valid source of information.

10. Do not hold in any natural body urges — such as crying, sneezing, peeing, yawning, or pooping — as they will cause pressure, blockages, or the development of abnormal passages.

11. Hold an intention and enjoy the process, but don't expect an outcome. You might get something better than you expected, so you don't want to miss that when it happens.

12. Encourage your partner to focus on his health, but don't try to do it for him.

13. Keep studying yourself, always.

Well-being comes from using your senses and intellect to make good decisions in the moment, while also having an awareness of the bigger contextual picture — the time of day, the seasons of the year, and the phase and conditions of your life. Each decision affects you in both the short and long term. If you have integrity in your decision-making, then your choices can actually allow you to operate in life more effectively, by both being in the moment and guiding yourself toward a better place. It is worthwhile for you to focus on rasayanas, or the ways *you* can have your best health, because it is better for everyone else in your world, including a possible future child.

Moving Forward

If you want to have a child, you must first start with making your own life healthy, wonderful, and beautiful. Your partner should do the same thing, and then the two of you can move forward together on your journey with clarity, integrity, healthy bodies, and healthy minds. This isn't a onetime thing that happens. It is an ongoing process if you want to have a great life.

Learn more about Ayurveda whenever you are interested in tapping into the primal nature of your being. The world is full of intellectual stimulation and mental distractions, but your body is tangible, an animal that has both stories to tell and urges that need to be listened to. Ayurveda taps you back into listening to your body and giving it what it needs. As you know, your body is very intelligent. It's doing way more to operate your life than your conscious mind is in any given moment. At the same time, it's your conscious mind that is going to help you move forward to improve your health.

Learn through your senses about the quality of your tissues, your particular doshas, the state of your agni, and all your excretions. These are your basic animal functions. Each tissue of your body has a specific purpose and function. Your reproductive health is a big indicator of your overall stamina and immunity. If this becomes compromised, it's not just reproductive capabilities that are at risk.

Get your intellect on board with the ways of nature. Learn how foods, spices, and herbs affect you. Learn how you challenge, nourish, or rough up your body and what that does to it. Remember your vulnerable spots so you can take good care of them. You can focus on yourself without losing sight of nature and the people around you.

This book outlines some protocols and practices you can explore to optimize your health and tap into the primal power of creation in a way that also sets you up for success later. Set your intentions for prepping your body, mind, and spirit for a healthy conception. Understand the basic Ayurvedic concepts and principles laid out in these pages. Use the self-assessment tools provided to determine your imbalance patterns and dominant dosha(s). Test your agni by trying the fasting experiment. Practice the protocols outlined in chapter 8 that apply to your imbalance patterns. Stick with these protocols for at least three to six months. Refine your practice by deepening your understanding of how food and sensory input can possibly affect you through the five elements and three doshas. Meanwhile, observe your partner's health, and notice how the two of you are doing together. Cleanse with an expert if you need more detoxification.

Once you are on the Ayurvedic path, even if it feels like you've taken only a small step, it always helps reinforce your new-and-improved direction by filling your life with people, objects, and events that remind you of your intentions. This is where building an altar at home or work comes in as an opportunity to provide a daily reminder.

Looking around you, you see the macrocosm, and inside you is the microcosm. Your network of people either support you in your forward journey or keep you clinging to the past. Fill your calendar with beneficial activities (or even open space) to design for your desired lifestyle. If you are unsure about your environment's ability to further your intentions, then a support group or some sort of educational program can be helpful. In all cases, you are being asked to step up to the plate, to be the most amazing version of yourself you can be.

I know that if you do a really good job implementing the health-promoting tools I've outlined in this book, you will probably expect to immediately get pregnant from them. However, I want to challenge you to not expect to get pregnant. Instead, I want you to focus on being your healthiest, happiest, most beautiful self, and discover what nature has in store for you. If Mother Nature wants *you* to be a mother, then she will let you know in very mysterious ways.

In every moment, you are being groomed to live the life you were meant to live in that moment. The life you think you are supposed to have is fiction. The life you don't want is fiction. The life you have right now — that is what's real.

This is the surrender we are all seeking, and it's right under our noses.

Acknowledgments

I want to thank:

The father of my child, Dr. David Lieberman, for being crazy enough to get me pregnant, and precise enough to do it on the first try.

Georgia Hughes and New World Library.

My parents, Dave's parents, and anyone else who has watched over my son so I could take the time to write and share this book.

My teachers and administrators from Mount Madonna Institute, especially Dr. Sarita Shrestha, Drs. Suhas and Manisha Kshirsagar, Dr. Vivek Shanbhag, Dr. Ram Harsh Singh, Dr. Vasant Lad, Dr. John Douillard, Kamalesh Hooven, Della Davis, Savita Brownfield, Sarada Diffenbaugh, and those from all the yoga teacher trainings throughout the years.

My clients and students, for getting wildly open with me.

Alexandra Kostoulas and Sasha Bravin, for guidance on writing and publishing.

Sanjay Soni, for brutal honesty.

Friends and colleagues who encouraged me to follow my passion when I was filled with doubt, especially Teresa Piro, Sarah Kucera, Jenna Furnari, Petra Neiger, Dr. Yi Chiang, Dr. Ana Dubey, Ravi Bhaskaran, Chitra Rajeshwari, Sally Mitchell, Keren Flavell, Dr. Neale Martin, and Aaron Wilkins.

Harmonia Wellness Center and Social Club, Sausalito, California; The Mindful Body; San Francisco, California; and Body Temp Yoga, San Francisco, California.

My former lovers — for all the practice.

Glossary of Sanskrit and Other Uncommon Terms

abhyanga — a body treatment involving the application of oil in massage-like strokes to the skin and underlying tissues to move doshas and ama into the detoxification channels of the body; a pacification treatment for vata.

agni — the digestive fire of the body, tissues, and individual cells; the fire god from ancient Vedic literature.

ahita — harmful to your health.

akasha — ether, or space; the first of the five elements of nature.

ama — the by-product of incomplete or improper digestion; a toxin that clogs the channels of the body and is one of the underlying causes of disease.

apana vayu — the downward-moving wind current of the body, governed by surrender to gravity.

artava — the female reproductive tissues that the ovum is released into and washed out of the body with.

asantarpana — a category of therapies in Ayurveda considered not nourishing, though they can still be beneficial.

asatmendriyartha samyoga — a misuse of the sense organs; one of the three main causes of disease.

Ashtanga Hrdayam — the second of the three major ancient texts on Ayurvedic medicine.

atman — the soul or spirit that is beyond material form and understanding.

Ayurveda — the science of life; life knowledge; a form of complementary medicine from the Indian subcontinent that teaches how optimal health is achieved when one lives in line with the principles of nature.

brahmacharya — the yogic practice of holding back one's sexual energy in order to master it.

brahmana — building therapy; one of the six major therapeutic measures in Ayurveda.

buddha — one who has achieved an enlightened state; one who has intellect.

chakras — the body's seven main energy centers, which are oriented along the spinal column, from the base of the spine to the crown of the head.

Charaka-samhita — the first of the three major ancient texts on Ayurvedic medicine.

dhatu — one of the seven main tissue types of the body, in which each cell has a common purpose and function.

doshas — functional humors of the body that can go out of balance due to issues of mind, body, and environment; when literally translated, *dosha* means "that which can go out of balance."

ghee — clarified butter; an oily substance derived from cow's milk that is eaten to nourish and lubricate the body and is delivered as a soothing agent in Ayurvedic body therapies.

gunas — attributes or qualities found in all of nature. Ayurveda defines ten pairs of opposite qualities (total of twenty) used to balance doshas.

hita — beneficial to your health.

jala — water; the fourth of the five elements of nature.

kala parinama — not being in line with the cycles of nature; not respecting the natural changes that occur due to the passage of time.

Kama-sutra — a classic Indian text on the numerous methods of sexual intercourse.

kapalabhati pranayama — a breathing practice for either decreasing kapha dosha or increasing udana vayu; when literally translated means "skull-shining breath."

kapha — the water and earth humor of the body, responsible for stability and lubrication; growth property.

khavaigunya — an injured, weak, or defective space in the body that is a place where doshas and ama can accumulate when imbalances occur.

kshetra — the field; a place where a person may take a pilgrimage.

kundalini — the primal, serpent energy that is either dormant at the base of the spine or activated and moving upward.

langhana — lightening therapy; one of the six major therapeutic measures in Ayurveda.

mastaka granthi — the head knot; a point located at the base of the skull, where the neck and head come together.

nadis — subtle channels in the body that energy travels through.

nidana parivargana — "to remove the cause of a disease."

ojas — that which provides immunity; the subtle essence of kapha that is the product of good nutrition and healthy agni.

om — a sacred syllable used as a simple mantra.

pitta — the fire and water humor of the body, responsible for transformation and heat; inflammation property.

prajnaparadha — "a crime of the intellect/wisdom"; the top cause of all disease.

prakruti — one's original and natural form that was created at conception.

prana — energy or life force.

prana vayu — the wind current of the body increased by breathing.

pranayama — breathing practice; controlling energy.

prithvi — earth; the fifth of the five elements of nature.

purvarupa — a warning sign that a dosha is getting out of balance.

rasayana — the therapeutic discipline of building good-quality tissues and strong immunity.

ritusandhi — the time when two seasons come together, providing good opportunities for rebalancing.

rukshana — roughening therapy; one of the six major therapeutic measures in Ayurveda.

rupa — an actual symptom of a dosha being out of balance.

samana vayu — the wind current of the body that equalizes the transfer of energy and nutrients between its inside and outside spaces.

samskara — an imprint left on the mind from an experience.

sattva — a clear state of mind in which one makes wholesome decisions

sheetali pranayama — a cooling breathing practice for pitta dosha.

shukra — male semen, which contains sperm.

snehana — oiling therapy; one of the six major therapeutic measures in Ayurveda.

stambhana — tightening therapy; one of the six major therapeutic measures in Ayurveda.

Sushruta-samhita — the third of the three major ancient texts of Ayurvedic medicine.

swedana — sweating therapy; one of the six major therapeutic measures in Ayurveda.

tejas — fire; the third of the five elements of nature.

udana vayu — the wind current of the body that moves from the gut to the head to facilitate thinking and communication.

ujjayi pranayama — a warming, focused breathing practice for kapha dosha; when literally translated means "victorious breath."

upavāsa — fasting; when literally translated means "to stay close to one's soul."

vajikarana — the therapeutic discipline of promoting or enhancing fertility in a depleted person.

vata — the air and space humor of the body, responsible for movement and change; degeneration property.

vayu — air; the second of the five elements of nature.

vinyasa yoga — a style of modern physical yoga practice that involves linking poses together in a sequence.

vyana vayu — the wind current of the body that circulates to and from its periphery due to the heart's pumping action.

yoga — to yoke together; a connected state.

yoga nidra — a style of yoga that involves the relaxation of the body through awareness exercises and no movement; when literally translated means "connected sleep."

Yoga-sutras — one of the classic texts on yoga philosophy and psychology, compiled prior to 400 CE by Patanjali and followed by yoga practitioners worldwide today; a book that describes how the mind operates and how to transcend thought waves.

Notes

Foreword

p. xii   *In a study of more than 8,800 women and 6,200 men*: Jessica Datta et al., "Prevalence of Infertility and Help Seeking among 15,000 Women and Men," *Human Reproduction* 31, no. 9 (September 2016): 218–18, https://www.ncbi.nlm.nih.gov/pmc/articles/PMC4991655.

p. xii   *Studies support the ancient wisdom of pregnancy preparation*: Mary E. Coussons-Read, "Effects of Prenatal Stress on Pregnancy and Human Development: Mechanisms and Pathways," *Obstetric Medicine* 6, no. 2 (June 2013): 52–57, https://www.ncbi.nlm.nih.gov/pmc/articles/PMC5052760.

p. xii   *In one study, 40 percent of women with infertility*: Kristin L. Rooney and Alice D. Domar, "The Relationship between Stress and Infertility," *Dialogues in Clinical Neuroscience* 20, no. 1 (March 2018): 41–47, https://www.ncbi.nlm.nih.gov/pmc/articles/PMC6016043.

p. xii   *in a study of 600 female physicians*: Natalie Clark Stentz, Kent A. Griffith, Elena Perkins, Rochelle DeCastro Jones, and Reshma Jagsi, "Fertility and Childbearing Among American Female Physicians," *Journal of Women's Health* 25, no. 10 (October 2016): 1059–65, https://www.liebertpub.com/doi/10.1089/jwh.2015.5638.

P. xiii   *once a woman is diagnosed with infertility, her levels of stress*: Rooney and Domar, "The Relationship between Stress and Infertility."

p. xiii   *Counseling to reduce infertility-related stress*: Rooney and Domar, "The Relationship between Stress and Infertility."

p. xiii   *have been shown to boost oxytocin*: Kerstin Uvnäs-Moberg, Linda Handlin, and Maria Petersson, "Self-Soothing Behaviors with Particular Reference to Oxytocin Release Induced by Non-noxious Sensory

Stimulation," *Frontiers in Psychology* 5 (January 2015): 1529, https://www
.ncbi.nlm.nih.gov/pmc/articles/PMC4290532.

p. xiv   *Many studies link lack of sattva*: Alessandro Ilacqua, Giulia Izzo, Gian
Pietro Emerenziani, Carlo Baldari, and Antonio Aversa, "Lifestyle and
Fertility: The Influence of Stress and Quality of Life on Male Fertility,"
Reproductive Biology and Endocrinology 16, no. 1 (November 2018): 115,
https://www.ncbi.nlm.nih.gov/pmc/articles/PMC6260894.

p. xiv   *There are four main types of rasayana used traditionally*: Vasant Lad,
Textbook of Ayurveda, vol. 3 (Albuquerque: Ayurvedic Press, 2012), 408;
and see my article "What Is Rasayana? Ayurvedic's Sacred Longevity
Therapies," November 14, 2019, https://lifespa.com/rasayana-longevity.

p. xv   *Classic behavioral rasayanas also include*: See also Douillard, "What Is
Rasayana?"

Introduction: How This Book Came About

p. 1   *"Creativity…begins in darkness"*: Julia Cameron, *The Artist's Way: A
Spiritual Path to Higher Creativity* (New York: Penguin, 1992), 194.

Chapter 1. Fertility Today

p. 7   *"Do not kill the instinct…"*: Vanda Scaravelli, *Awakening the Spine: The
Stress-Free New Yoga That Works with the Body to Restore Health, Vitality
and Energy* (San Francisco: HarperSanFrancisco, 1991), 38.

p. 9   *The number of childless women*: Gretchen Livingston and D'Vera Cohn,
"Childlessness Up Among All Women; Down Among Women with Advanced Degrees," Social & Demographic Trends, Pew Research Center,
June 25, 2010, http://www.pewsocialtrends.org/2010/06/25/childlessness
-up-among-all-women-down-among-women-with-advanced-degrees.

p. 9   *the average woman in the world*: "Fertility Rate, Total (Births per
Woman)," Data, The World Bank, accessed June 16, 2019, http://data
.worldbank.org/indicator/SP.DYN.TFRT.IN.

p. 9   *women in global areas of conflict*: "Fertility Rate."

p. 11   *more than half of American workers*: "State of American Vacation 2018,"
Project: Time Off, U.S. Travel Association, online survey conducted
January 4–23, 2018, http://www.ustravel.org/sites/default/files/media_root
/document/2018_Research_State%20of%20American%20Vacation%20
2018.pdf.

p. 11   *A high percentage of people*: "Stress in America: The State of Our Nation,"
American Psychological Association, November 1, 2017, http://www.apa
.org/news/press/releases/stress/2017/state-nation.pdf.

p. 13   *12.6 being the mean age*: Anjani Chandra et al., "Fertility, Family Planning, and Reproductive Health of U.S. Women: Data From the 2002
National Survey of Family Growth," *Vital and Health Statistics*, series 23,
no. 25 (December 2005), National Center for Health Statistics, Centers
for Disease Control, Hyattsville, MD, https://www.cdc.gov/nchs/data
/series/sr_23/sr23_025.pdf.

p. 20   *Only 17 percent of women*: William D. Mosher, Anjani Chandra, and
Jo Jones, "Sexual Behavior and Selected Health Measures: Men and
Women 15–44 Years of Age, United States, 2002," *Advance Data From
Vital and Health Statistics*, no. 362 (September 15, 2005), National Center
for Health Statistics, Centers for Disease Control, Hyattsville, MD,
http://www.cdc.gov/nchs/data/ad/ad362.pdf.

p. 20   *The teenager of the modern society*: Joyce A. Martin et al., "Births: Final
Data for 2016," *National Vital Statistics Reports* 67, no. 1 (January 31,
2018), National Center for Health Statistics, Centers for Disease Control, Hyattsville, MD, http://www.cdc.gov/nchs/data/nvsr/nvsr67
/nvsr67_01.pdf.

p. 21   *As of 2012, less than 50 percent*: Lindsay M. Monte and Renee R. Ellis,
"Fertility of Women in the United States: 2012," U.S. Census Bureau,
July 2014, http://www.census.gov/content/dam/Census/library
/publications/2014/demo/p20-575.pdf.

p. 25   *It happens in about 5 percent of women*: Jan L. Shifren and Margery L. S.
Gass, "The North American Menopause Society Recommendations for
Clinical Care of Midlife Women," *Menopause* 21, no. 10 (October 2014):
1038–62, https://doi.org/10.1097/gme.000000000000319.

Chapter 2. Going Primal

p. 27   *"Let your mind go…"*: *L.A. Story*, directed by Mick Jackson, written by
Steve Martin (TriStar Pictures, 1991).

p. 28   *Yogananda believed that upon conception*: Swami Kriyananda, *Conversations with Yogananda*, 1st ed. (Nevada City, CA: Crystal Clarity Publish-
ers, 2004), 206.

Chapter 3. Principles of Health

p. 39   *"I believe it's really about unfolding ourselves"*: *The Feminine Unfolding*,
performance by Angela Farmer, 1999.

p. 42   *"A person with [a] uniformly healthy digestion…"*: Kaviraj Kunjalal
Bhishagratna, trans., ed., *Suśruta Saṃhitā*: Text with English Translation, a Full and Comprehensive Introduction, Additional Text, Different

Readings, Notes, Comparative Views, Index, Glossary and Plates (Varanasi, India: Chowkhamba Sanskrit Series Office, 1998), 140.

p. 55   *"Humans are not sleeping…"*: Matthew P. Walker, *Why We Sleep: Unlocking the Power of Sleep and Dreams* (New York: Scribner, 2018), 68.

Chapter 4. The Four Fertility Factors

p. 63   *"The upwelling of the sea continues"*: Brenda Hillman, "A Spiral Tries to Feel Again," *Seasonal Works with Letters on Fire* (Middletown, CT: Wesleyan University Press, 2013), 48.

p. 66   *as only 3 percent*: L. Rynn, J. Cragan, and A. Correa, "Update on Overall Prevalence of Major Birth Defects — Atlanta, Georgia, 1978–2005," *MMWR Weekly* 57, no. 1 (January 11, 2008): 1–5, National Center on Birth Defects and Developmental Disabilities, Centers for Disease Control and Prevention, Atlanta, GA, http://www.cdc.gov/mmwr/preview /mmwrhtml/mm5701a2.htm.

p. 69   *Their children are at greater risk*: Dan Shan et al., "Pregnancy Outcomes in Women of Advanced Maternal Age: A Retrospective Cohort Study from China," *Scientific Reports* 8, article no. 12239 (August 16, 2018), https://doi.org/10.1038/s41598-018-29889-3.

p. 88   *caffeine applied to the skin*: Nina Otberg et al., "The Role of Hair Follicles in the Percutaneous Absorption of Caffeine," *British Journal of Clinical Pharmacology* 65, no. 4 (April 2008), 488–92, https://bpspubs .onlinelibrary.wiley.com/doi/full/10.1111/j.1365-2125.2007.03065.x.

Chapter 5. Discovering Your Type

p. 93   *"According to Ayurveda…"*: Vasant Lad, *Ayurveda: The Science of Self-Healing: A Practical Guide* (Twin Lakes, WI: Lotus Press, 1985), 29.

p. 101   *Not following the circadian rhythm*: Fiona C. Baker and Helen S. Driver, "Circadian Rhythms, Sleep, and the Menstrual Cycle," *Sleep Medicine* 8, no. 6 (October 2007), 613–22, https://doi.org/10.1016/j.sleep.2006.09.011.

p. 102   *Since 55 percent of Americans*: Teresa Carr, "Too Many Meds? America's Love Affair with Prescription Medication," *Consumer Reports*, August 3, 2017, http://www.consumerreports.org/prescription-drugs/too-many -meds-americas-love-affair-with-prescription-medication.

Chapter 6. Engaging the Heart

p. 113   *"You are the instrument…"*: Rama Jyoti Vernon, *Yoga: The Practice of Myth and Sacred Geometry*, 1st ed. (Twin Lakes, WI: Lotus Press, 2014), 11.

Chapter 7. Learning How to Read Your Body

p. 123   *"Woman is the source of creation"*: Dr. Sarita Shrestha, "Disease Management: Women's Health Issues," class, Mount Madonna Institute, Watsonville, CA, May 2, 2014.

p. 124   *Ayurveda's Indicators of Fertility*: P. V. Sharma, Caraka Saṃhitā, vol. II (Varanasi, India: Chaukhambha Orientalia, 2014), 423.

p. 134   *both body temperature and level of physical activity*: Trevor T. Nyakudya et al., "Body Temperature and Physical Activity Correlates of the Menstrual Cycle in Chacma Baboons (*Papio hamadryas ursinus*)," *American Journal of Primatology* 74, no. 12 (December 2012): 1143–53, https://doi .org/10.1002/ajp.22073.

p. 137   *men who ejaculate less frequently*: Brent M. Hanson et al., "The Impact of Ejaculatory Abstinence on Semen Analysis Parameters: A Systematic Review," *Journal of Assisted Reproduction and Genetics* 35, no. 2 (February 2018): 213–20, https://doi.org/10.1007/s10815-017-1086-0.

p. 137   *men's sperm counts have collectively decreased*: Hagai Levine et al., "Temporal Trends in Sperm Count: A Systematic Review and Meta-Regression Analysis," *Human Reproduction Update* 23, no. 6 (November 2017): 646–59, https://doi.org/10.1093/humupd/dmx022.

Chapter 8. Healing Fertility Rituals and Practices

p. 143   *"Our bodies are ideally designed…"*: Janet Balaskas, *Preparing for Birth with Yoga: Exercises for Pregnancy and Childbirth*, illustrated ed. (Rockport, MA: Element Books, 1994), 18.

p. 162   *a heightened sense of smell*: Evelia Navarrete-Palacios et al., "Lower Olfactory Threshold during the Ovulatory Phase of the Menstrual Cycle," *Biological Psychology* 63, no. 3 (July 2003): 269–79, https://doi.org/10.1016 /s0301-0511(03)00076-0.

p. 162   *being more sensitive to noise*: Meenal Batta et al., "Effect of Different Phases of Menstrual Cycle on Brainstem Auditory Evoked Response," *International Journal of Applied & Basic Medical Research* 7, no. 1 (January–March 2017): 44–47, https://doi.org/10.4103/2229-516X.198522.

Chapter 9. Your Partner

p. 179   *"You make love differently…"*: Wendy Doniger, *Redeeming the Kamasutra*, 1st ed. (New York: Oxford University Press, 2016), 22–23.

p. 190   *"thick, sweet, unctuous…"*: P. V. Sharma, Caraka Saṃhitā, vol. II (Varanasi, India: Chaukhambha Orientalia, 2014), 51.

p. 190   *Dry or scanty semen*: Sharma, 464, 474.

p. 192   *"a sexually excited female partner"*: Sharma, 35.

p. 196   *"Let the beauty we love…"*: Coleman Barks, trans., *The Essential Rumi* (Edison, NJ: Castle Books, 1997), 36.

Chapter 10. Your Environment

p. 197   *"And every breath we drew was Hallelujah"*: Leonard Cohen, "Hallelujah," *Various Positions* (New York: Columbia, 1984).

Index

About the Author

Heather Grzych is a board-certified Ayurvedic practitioner who bridges the worlds of conventional and alternative medicine to help women and men heal their physical and emotional lives. She is on the board of directors for the National Ayurvedic Medical Association and has consulted with doctors, governments, and insurance companies.

Heather tried unsuccessfully to get pregnant in her early thirties and credits Ayurveda with later helping her get pregnant on the first try and have a child just before turning forty. She regularly lectures at wellness centers and yoga studios in the San Francisco Bay Area and guides people through life-changing fasting and cleansing programs. Visit her website: heathergrzych.com.

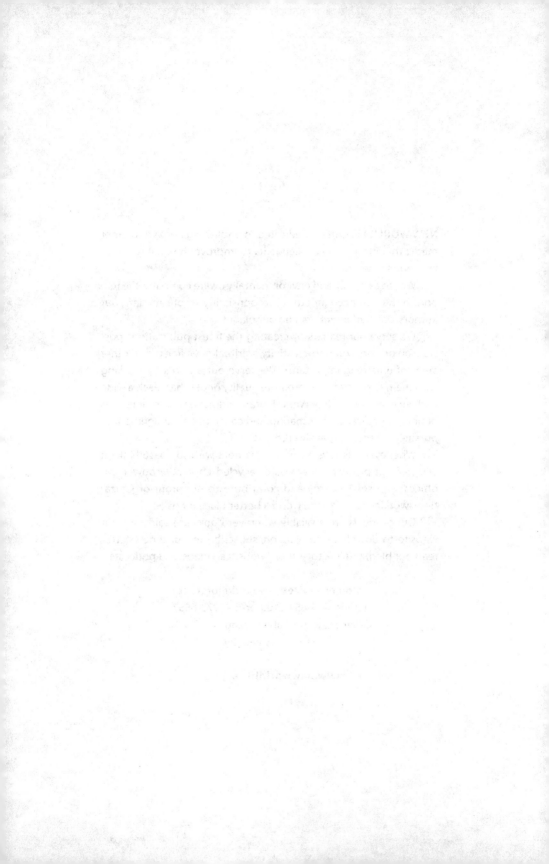